LEMON DIET

Step by step guide to detox your body and
lose weight with pleasure.
Lots of recipes to feel better and be more
healthy in a natural way.
How to eat healthy, lose weight and improve
your life with the lemon diet.

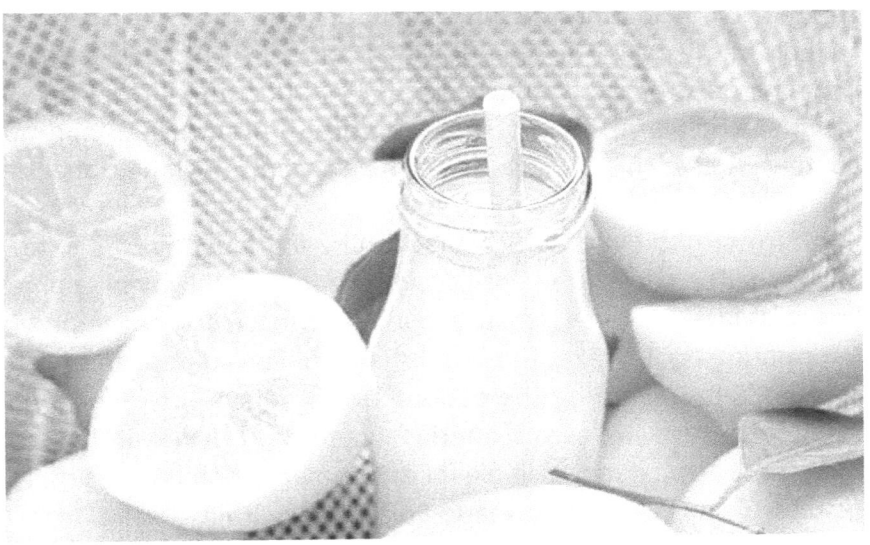

JARD RAWLINS

TABLE OF CONTENTS

Introduction

First of all I want to thank you for purchasing a copy of the Lemon Diet. The human's being nature, especially in today's society, is to find a quick and easy solution to any problem that may arise. This is especially true when it comes to physical appearance. Following a diet consistently and firmly is not an easy task, and it is inevitable that a lot of immediate and productive methods will be sought in order to get back into shape in the blink of an eye, especially if we consider that summer has arrived, and no one likes to feel uncomfortable in a swimsuit, regardless of weight. And this is where the lemon diet comes to our rescue. It is a diet which needs to be followed for a maximum of one month, which not only promises a "detox" effect for our body, but also a rapid and effective slimming. So, if you are trying to lose a few extra pounds quickly, or even just that minimum to get along well with yourself regarding the upcoming costume test, the lemon diet might be the ideal solution to the problem. This diet makes you lose weight faster than the average and makes the body regain its balance and above all the organs undergo a "purification" process. Studies have shown that when the body detoxifies, the skin becomes smoother and more radiant, and blemishes such as acne, wrinkles and spots caused by free radicals in our body are also reduced. In addition to the multiple benefits offered by this diet, we must also consider the risks that it may or may not involve. First, given the low assortment of foods you can consume, following this diet could lead to harmful consequences such as poor concentration, mood swings and a feeling of fatigue and weakness. Furthermore, like any diet that promises to lose weight in a short time, if followed for too long, you may be more inclined to quickly recover all the lost pounds. During the course of the diet you can have a deficiency of vitamins and minerals. In that case you must immediately stop following it and return to a normal diet. Prolonged use of lemon juice can also cause enamel damage to our teeth. It is important to always be careful with this type of diet and learn to read the signals the body sends to us so that we can take the right precautions in case of need.

Historical notes

The origin of lemon is still unclear, although it is likely to think that the first trees grew in Assam (a region in Northeastern India), in Northern Burma and in China. A genetic study on the origin of lemon has concluded that it could be a hybrid between bitter orange and cedar.

The lemons were known in the Jewish religion from ancient times, according to Giuseppe Flavio (Roman historian), they used them to attack a wandering priest during the festival of 90 BC. In Europe the lemons arrive from the south of Italy in the first century AD (at the time of ancient Rome); however, they did not immediately arouse great interest. Later they arrived in Persia and then in Iraq and Egypt around 700 AD. Here, the first evidence of the lemon was recorded in a tenth century Arab agricultural treatise. The lemon could both be eaten and used as an ornament in the first Islamic gardens. In the following years it was distributed throughout the Arab and Mediterranean territory starting from 1000 until 1150 AD. The first cultivation known in Italy was made in the Genoa area.

The lemon was introduced to America in 1493, when Christopher Columbus brought the lemon seeds of "Hispaniola" during his journeys of discovery. Spanish patrons in America have helped bring lemon seeds to the other side of the globe. In America, lemon was initially used as an ornamental and medicinal plant. In 1747 James Lind added lemon juice to the sailors' diet suffering from scurvy, although for obvious reasons vitamin C was not yet known. In the nineteenth century, in California and Florida, the first lemon citrus groves appeared. The origin of the word "lemon" should be Middle Eastern. We talk about lemons in an English customs document dating back to 1420-1421.

Lemon and its cultivation

The lemon (Citrus limonum) is an evergreen plant of the Rutaceae family native from East Asia.

The lemon tree is a plant of medium height with perennial, alternate and ovate leaves.

The lemon fruit has a wrinkled skin, formed by an outer layer called flavedo, thin and yellow in which are found the glands full of essential oil, and an inner layer called albedo ehich is white, thick and bitter.

The inside of the fruit is divided into segments, from eight to ten, covered with thin membranes, containing the seeds and numerous vesicles rich in acid juice and particular substances important for numerous metabolic activities of the human body. In ideal conditions, the plant is in continuous bloom.

Lemon prefers warm and not windy climates. In Italy, the largest production comes from Sicily and then from Calabria, Campania and Puglia.

Numerous protected geographical indications (PGIs) of lemons grown in particularly suitable Italian productive areas have been recognized at European level, namely:

- in Sicily the Syracuse PGI lemon and the interdonato lemon PGI;
- in Calabria the Rocca Imperiale IGP lemon;
- in Campania, the Costa d'Amalfi PGI lemon and the IGP Sorrento lemon;
- in Puglia the lemon of the Gargano PGI.

These are the main ones.

How to grow potted lemons

Lemons, how to grow them? If you have at your disposal organic lemons, a garden, a large balcony or a terrace, you could try to grow this small citrus plant in a pot, which is well suited for the warm climate. Growing lemons in pots requires a few tricks, but it can give a great satisfaction, starting from the possibility of having fresh and fragrant fruits always available.

You can choose to bury one of the seeds in a seedbed or directly in a round pot with a diameter of about 30 centimeters, filled with well-draining soil and a saucer underneath. The ideal temperature for germination is around

15 degrees. The germination period could be extended from 1 to 2 months, and even longer, depending on the climate and outside temperature. It is therefore necessary to be patient and water your pot regularly, keeping the surface of the soil moist. It is advisable to use a spray container.

How to grow a lemon tree

In the first period the plant must be watered daily, the soil needs to be kept always damp, while, at the same time, the formation of water stagnation in the saucer needs to be avoided, which could compromise the resistance of the roots. Once the seedling has become sufficiently robust and has reached a height of at least 15-20 centimeters, repotting can be done.

Where to place the lemon plant

The compost can be added to the soil at a rate of 10%. It is advisable to avoid plastic vases and prefer stone or terracotta garden pots, so that the plant does not suffer. The vase must be placed in an area which is sunny and sheltered from air stream. For this reason we usually tend to place the vase at a short distance from the external bulkheads of the house, along one of the sunny sides.

It is important to shelter the lemon tree when it faces its first winter. Younger plants need plenty of light during the day and a temperature of not less than 12 degrees. In any case, the excessively heated interior spaces of the house and the placement of the lemon pot in the vicinity of entrance doors or radiators must be avoided. Your lemon plant should be guaranteed an exposure to sunlight of at least 6-8 hours a day, especially during the warm season.

When to change the pot of the lemon tree

Repotting will take place every two years and during the growth of the plant it will be possible to proceed with pruning, so that its foliage can take on the desired shape. In other cases, it may be allowed to grow freely. The ideal period for repotting is the beginning of spring, especially during March. The transfer of the pot from outside to inside, or vice versa, depending on the season, must be done in a manner as gradual as possible, in order to prevent the plant from suffering. The ideal pruning period is the end of winter, so that the plant will be ready to regenerate with the arrival of spring. In the case of adult plants, the repotting can be reduced up to four years. It is important to adjust to the diameter of the vase, keeping in mind that it must correspond to the expansion of the foliage of the lemon tree. An adult plant can require a vase with a diameter of 80 centimeters. Once these dimensions are reached, the repotting can be considered definitive. The lemon trees grown in pots tend to suffer more from both drought and cold, which is why it is so important to take care of their correct positioning throughout the year.

Seed plants have fewer fruits than grafted plants. However, this is not a strict rule. As well as we know, it is nature that dictates the times of flowering and fruit ripening. In order to enjoy many fruits in just a few years, it is usually recommended to perform a graft. The best time for grafting is spring. During flowering the plant must be watered often, in order to avoid the risk of ruining the leaves. The presence of yellow leaves is an indication of insufficient watering, so you can adjust accordingly. Lemon trees are actually delicate, but with the right care and attention they can accompany you for years with their fresh fruits and their unmistakable scent.

Lemon-based slimming drinks

Hot water and lemon cocktail

Ingredients
3 untreated lemons
600 ml of water
honey to taste
parsley to taste

Preparation
Put 3 lemons cut in half in 600 ml of water in a saucepan and leave to boil for about 3 minutes. When the mixture has cooled, remove the lemons and drink a cup on an empty stomach every morning. The doses indicated are sufficient for 2 or 3 days. The drink can be kept in the fridge. It can be consumed cold and reheated before being taken. To have it a little sweeter add a teaspoon of honey to taste. Parsley is also a valuable aid to purify and facilitate weight loss thanks to its active ingredients that help digestion and promote the drainage of liquids. Parsley can be added directly in a cup or in pieces to enrich and garnish. To get the greatest benefits, water and lemon should be drunk for 5 consecutive days in the morning before breakfast. Allow at least another 10 days before resuming administration.

The cocktail of water and lemon not only helps to detoxify and lose weight but also brings other important benefits. It is considered a real elixir of long life. It contains large amounts of vitamin C and mineral salts, such as potassium, magnesium and calcium, considered fundamental for psycho-physical well-being. It helps the immune defenses and especially when there is flu or cold.

Detoxifying and purifying drink for the body

Ingredients
100 g of celery
50 g of fennel
5 g of fennel seeds
200 g of apples
1 tablespoon of aloe vera juice
1 piece of ginger
1 piece of untreated lemon

Preparation
Boil the fennel seeds to soften them up. Wash the celery, fennel and apples. Cut them into pieces. Peel half a lemon and set it aside. Peel a piece of fresh ginger. Centrifuge the celery, apple, fennel, ginger, lemon and the fennel seeds soaked in order to extract the juices. It is advisable to use a centrifuge capable of extracting cold juices to prevent the active ingredients from rapid oxidation. Add the aloe vera juice to the obtained mixture and immediately consume it in order to prevent the oxidation of the active ingredients and keep their properties unaltered.

Slimming lemonade

Ingredients

30 cl of water
2 tablespoons of lemon juice
2 tablespoons of maple syrup
A pinch of cayenne pepper

Preparation

Boil 30 cl of water with 2 tablespoons of lemon juice. After turning off the heat, add 2 tablespoons of maple syrup and a pinch of cayenne pepper. Let cool for a few minutes before pouring the liquid into a cup.

The lemonade obtained must be drunk several times during the day:

- as soon as you wake up
- after the mid-morning and mid-afternoon snack
-before going to sleep.

To get the greatest possible benefits, lemonade should be taken for several consecutive days alternating with a few days off.

Water, lemon and ginger tea

Ingredients
a cup of water
a slice of fresh ginger or half a teaspoon of grated ginger
lemon juice

Preparation
Warm up the water paying attention that it does not boil. Add the ginger (sliced or grated) and let stand for 5 minutes. Remove from heat and add the lemon juice. The herbal tea is ready. It is preferably drunk in the morning and in the evening but it can also cheer up the mid-day breaks.

Digestive decoction with lemon and laurel (canary)

Ingredients

Water

1 untreated lemon

Bay leaves

Preparation

Boil the water in a small pan and add the peel of the untreated lemon and the bay leaves.

Leave to infuse for 15 minutes and then let it rest for another ten minutes.

Strain and pour into a cup.

This infusion is also known as "Canary" due to the yellow color of the lemon peel.

It is recommended to drink this infusion in order to facilitate digestion.

Lemon and cinnamon infusion

Ingredients
1 cup of water (250 ml)
5 tablespoons of lemon juice (50 ml)
a cinnamon stick
1 teaspoon of honey (7.5 g)

Preparation
Heat the water and when it begins to boil add the cinnamon and honey. Leave to infuse for a quarter of an hour and then let it rest for another ten minutes. Strain and pour into a cup. Add 5 tablespoons of lemon juice. Drink the infusion every day on an empty stomach. Cinnamon and lemon is useful in treating arthritis by exerting a beneficial action in reducing inflammation and swelling. If you take the herbal tea 20 minutes after the main meal of the day, the cinnamon and lemon will help to the disposal of the most resistant fat which settles on the abdominal area, leading to weight loss.

Benefits of water and lemon intake

- It has a detox effect and has a purifying action (it is an excellent diuretic)
- Helps to lose weight and has a draining action
- Reduces inflammation
- Strengthens the immune system
- Helps digestion
- Keeps the skin beautiful and radiant
- Influences nail health
- Improves gum health
- It is an excellent source of vitamins, mineral salts and trace elements
- It is a source of energy
- Improves mood
- Helps balancing the body's PH levels
- Promotes the elimination of uric acid
- Promotes wound healing
- Refresh breath
- Hydrates and improves the lymphatic system
- Fights the flu
- Helps circulation
- Positively affects lowering of pressure
- Has an antioxidant action
- Has an anti-inflammatory and anticancer action
- Prevents kidney stones
- Has a digestive action
- Has an antiseptic action
- Lemon is a natural antibiotic and antibacterial that stimulates white blood cells to take action in order to defend the body.

The nutritional properties of Lemon

100 grams of lemon provide:

    Energy: 45 Kcal
    Water: 85 grams
    Lipids: 0.6 grams
    Potassium: 149 mg
    Calcium: 11 mg
    Vitamin C: 11 mg (71% of what an adult needs)
    Magnesium: 28 mg

Lemon diet

The lemon diet devised by Dr. Martine Andrè immediately became famous thanks to several public figures who declared they use it to lose weight and keep fit.

This diet is based on the consumption of lemon, a food with great draining and detoxifying effects able to accelerate the metabolism, thus favoring weight loss (up to 3 kilos per week).

A low calorie diet should be associated with the consumption of the drinks mentioned above, in which it is possible to take other foods during the day, mainly: yoghurt, fresh and dried fruit, oatmeal flakes, vegetable salad, whole wheat bread, soups, vegetables, avocado, fish, chicken breast, eggs, bread and whole wheat pasta.

Thanks again for choosing this book, make sure to leave a short review on Amazon if you enjoy it. I'd really love to hear your thoughts!

Scheme of the weekly menu

As an example, a weekly menu will be proposed below. If you want to experiment with this diet or lose weight, it is strongly recommended, however, to rely on a professional in order to have, in complete safety, a personalized plan tailored to your specific and real needs.

MONDAY
Breakfast: lemonade then about half an hour later yogurt (also a vegetable), 2 tablespoons of oat flakes and a fruit
Snack: fresh fruit and lemonade
Lunch: vegetable soup with wholemeal bread
Snack: dried fruit and lemonade
Dinner: fish with vegetables with lemon juice dressing
Before going to sleep: lemonade

TUESDAY
Breakfast: lemonade then about half an hour later fruit salad, barley coffee and some almonds
Snack: raw vegetables and lemonade
Lunch: lemon risotto
Snack: dried fruit and lemonade
Dinner: chicken breast with vegetables and lemon juice dressing
Before going to sleep: lemonade

WEDNESDAY
Breakfast lemonade then about half an hour later fruit salad and toast
Snack: fresh fruit and lemonade
Lunch: bean salad with vegetables and lemon juice dressing
Snack: fresh cheese, raw vegetables and lemonade
Dinner: omelet with vegetables and lemon juice dressing, and wholemeal bread
Before going to sleep: lemonade

THURSDAY

Breakfast: lemonade then about half an hour later oats, fruit and yogurt

Snack: a handful of almonds and lemonade

Lunch: whole wheat pasta with vegetables

Snack: fresh fruit and lemonade

Dinner: lentils, salad and wholemeal bread

Before going to sleep: lemonade

FRIDAY

Breakfast: lemonade then about half an hour later fresh fruit and wholemeal bread

Snack: raw vegetables and lemonade

Lunch: whole-wheat pasta with tuna and vegetables with lemon dressing

Snack: dried fruit and lemonade

Dinner: fish with vegetables and lemon juice dressing

Before going to sleep: lemonade

SATURDAY

Breakfast: lemonade then about half an hour later yogurt (also a vegetable), 2 tablespoons of oat flakes and a fruit

Snack: almonds and lemon juice

Lunch: toast and vegetable soup

Snack: fresh cheese and raw vegetables, lemonade

Dinner: white meat with vegetables seasoned with lemon juice

Before going to sleep: lemonade

SUNDAY

Breakfast: about half an hour before having breakfast, drink the lemonade then eat fruit salad seasoned with lemon

Snack: dried fruit and lemonade

Lunch: brown rice with vegetables

Snack: raw vegetables and lemonade

Dinner: low-fat cheese with vegetables and whole wheat bread

Before going to sleep: lemonade

Flash diet to detoxify the liver - 3 days

If you want to follow a detoxifying and deflating diet for up to 72 hours, you can follow a menu like the one indicated below. It is always good to remember to drink 1 liter of water and various herbal teas.

DAY 1
Breakfast: 1 cup of oatmeal with berries and oilseeds, or 3 hard-boiled eggs
Snack: 1 handful of raw almonds
Lunch: grilled chicken breast with boiled vegetables (beetroot, carrots, parsnips, green beans) seasoned with lemon + 1 tablespoon of unsalted almonds
Dinner: baked fish with boiled beans

DAY 2
Breakfast: 1 cup of oatmeal with seasonal fruit pieces and unsalted almonds
Snack: 1 seasonal fruit
Lunch: grilled zucchini seasoned with pepper, lemon, vinegar, thyme + grated carrot seasoned with olive oil, lemon and chopped parsley
Dinner: steamed vegetables or string beans and boiled broccoli seasoned with 1 tablespoon of olive oil

DAY 3
Breakfast: 1 cup of oatmeal with fresh seasonal fruit, oilseeds and 1 tablespoon of almonds
Snack: 1 handful of nuts or other dried fruit
Lunch: grilled chicken seasoned with rosemary, thyme and lemon juice or cooked with onions, black olives and thyme
Dinner: vegetable soup (mushrooms, onions, carrots, garlic, celery, bay leaves and thyme) with whole grains topped with 1 drop of oil

Light diet for weight loss - 1 day

If, on the other hand, you want to experiment with a simpler, one-day diet, you can take a menu like the one shown below as an example for a detoxifying diet, always remembering that it is strongly recommended to rely on a nutritionist.

In the morning on an empty stomach drink 1 lemon juice in 1 glass of warm water.
It detoxifies and stimulates the work of the liver.

Breakfast
1 mushed banana with 2 tablespoons of canola oil + 1 lemon juice. Mix well and add 3 pieces of seasonal fruit and 1 tablespoon of crushed oil seeds (almonds, walnuts, hazelnuts ...) or rusks.
1 herbal tea of bitter depurative herbs such as birch, artichoke, dandelion or cherry peduncles

Lunch
Mixed salad as an appetizer (or 1 glass of vegetable extract for those who do not tolerate raw vegetables well), dressed with 1 tablespoon of olive oil
1 fish fillet or 1 grilled chicken breast accompanied by cooked vegetables

Morning and afternoon snack
1 baked fruit or 1 raw seasonal fruit
1 herbal tea with draining herbs (queen of meadows, ash, birch)

Dinner
Vegetable soup, vegetables and whole grains, seasoned with 1 teaspoon of olive oil

The evening
1 purifying herbal tea, such as nettle, elderberry, horsetail and fennel

To drink
1 liter of water, better off meals

Contraindications

Like all flashy and fashionable diets, the one with lemon also has some drawbacks. Most of the time it is not balanced, it proposes a fast weight loss but with the possible risk to find oneself fighting with the yo-yo effect or the fact of regaining weight quickly once the diet is interrupted.

The real problem, however, is that it is a diet that does not provide proper nutrition education and therefore does not offer a healthy and long-lasting way of eating. Furthermore, if you follow it for too long, you may experience symptoms such as: fatigue, bad mood, lack of concentration, headaches and more.

The excessive use of lemon juice can eventually cause damage to tooth enamel, accentuate pre-existing gastritis and should be used with caution by those suffering from gastroesophageal reflux. It is strongly recommended that you rely on a nutritionist to have a balanced, healthy and effective diet which matches your needs.

Appetizers and Side Dishes

PEPPERED MUSSELS

Ingredients for 4 people
Mussels to be cleaned: 2 kg
Black pepper to be ground at the time q.b.
Parsley q.b.
Lemons q.b.

Preparation
We begin the preparation with the cleaning of the mussels. First of all make sure that they are all closed: the broken or open ones will have to be discarded. Remove the 'beard' - a fibrous clump of hairs that sprouts from the shell - by giving it a sharp tug towards the hinge end of the mussel. Place cleaned mussels in a fresh bowl of cold water until ready to use. Change this water two or three times to remove any salt or sand that the mussels may expel.

Rinse them thoroughly and move to the stove. Heat a very large pan, toss the mussels and immediately add the black pepper (better to grind the pepper at the moment, you will get a result with a more aromatic and intense taste).

Close with the lid and let the bivalves open completely. Occasionally shake the pot to stir. It will take 3-4 minutes. When cooked, remove the lid and place on the serving plates garnishing as desired with lemon wedges and chopped parsley.
The mussel is ready: good appetite!

OCTOPUS AND PARSLEY SALAD

Ingredients for 4 people
Octopus 850 g
Garlic 1 clove
Carrots 150 g
Celery 1 coast
Laurel 3 leaves
Black peppercorns 6
Salt 4 g
TO CONSIDER
Parsley 10 g
Extra virgin olive oil 30 g
Lemons 10 g
Salt 3 g
Black pepper 1 pinch

Preparation
To prepare the parsley octopus salad, start by cleaning the octopus: rinse it under running water, transfer it to a clean, dry cloth and pat dry with kitchen paper. Put it on a cutting board and with a knife cut the bag at eye level to eliminate it; also eliminate the beak, then hang the meat after beating with a hammer or a meat mallet. Rinse the octopus again under cold running water and remove the entrails from the bag by washing it carefully inside; wash and rub with your hands the head and tentacles to remove as much as possible patina that covers them.
Peel the carrot with a vegetable peeler, then cut it into small pieces together with the celery.
Place a large saucepan with water on the heat; pour the vegetables, bay leaves, garlic and add the pepper and salt.
When the water begins to boil, curl the tips of the octopus tentacles, immerse the tentacles in the boiling water and let them re-emerge. Continue like this for 4-5 times: in this way the preparation will be more pleasant. Then put the octopus in a pot and cook on very low heat for 30-35 minutes (about 20 minutes for every 500 g of octopus), covering with lid. Before draining it, stick the meat with a fork to check the cooking. When cooked, place it in a

bowl with water and ice for cooling. Transfer it onto a cutting board: with a knife separate the head from the tentacles, divide it in half, then cut the tentacles into small pieces, putting them in a small bowl. Squeeze a lemon and chop the parsley. Add the lemon juice and the chopped parsley to the octopus.

Season with oil, salt and pepper, then mix everything with a teaspoon. Your octopus salad is ready. Serve in a serving dish garnished with lemon slices.

ARTICHOKE, MUSHROOM AND BACON OMELET

Ingredients for 4 people

Eggs 6
Artichokes 5
Porcini or champignon mushrooms 200 g
Diced bacon 60 g
Milk 3 tablespoons
Garlic 1 clove
Chopped parsley 1 tbsp
Extra virgin olive oil 2 tbsp
Salt up to q.b.
Black pepper q.b.
Lemons 1
Grana Padano PDO 30 g

Preparation

To prepare the omelet with artichokes, mushrooms and smoked bacon, start by cleaning the artichokes watching the video of cooking school; you will only have to use hearts and stems. Clean the mushrooms and cut them into small pieces. Cut the artichoke hearts into thin slices and the stems into small pieces and keep them in acidulated water to prevent them from turning black. Fry a chopped clove of garlic and then add the diced bacon, rinsed and drained artichokes and chopped mushrooms. Add the chopped parsley and season with salt and pepper. Cook for 10 minutes. Meanwhile, in a bowl, beat the 6 eggs with a fork, add the grated Grana Padano and the milk and mix the ingredients.

When the vegetables are cooked, pour the mixture into the pan, stir immediately to mix the eggs and the vegetables and let the omelet thicken. Turn it when the bottom is cooked and cook it on the other side as well. We chose to serve the artichoke, mushroom and smoked bacon omelette as an appetizer, cutting it into squares.

ARTICHOKES WITH A STRINGY HEART

Ingredients for 4 people
Artichokes 1 kg

Montasio 65 g

Eggs 1

Parsley 12 g

Bread crumbs 300 g

Lemons 1

Grana Padano PDO to be grated 50 g

Garlic 1 clove

Salt up to q.b.

Black pepper q.b.

FOR BREADING
Eggs 2

Breadcrumbs 100 g

TO FRY
Seed oil q.b.

Montasio is a cheese from northern Italy with a Protected Designation of Origin. It is a typical Friulian cheese. It takes its name from the famous Montasio plateau, where cheese is produced since 1200, at the Abbey of Moggio Udinese.

It takes on a different taste, appearance, color and texture depending on the months of maturation. It is distinguished in fresh, medium and old. Depending on the seasoning it can take on a different flavor, the pasta is white and its crust is soft. As the seasoning increases, the flavor becomes more aromatic, the rind becomes harder, the color is more yellow and the soft dough becomes crumbly and hard.

Preparation
Start cleaning the artichokes: remove the outer leaves and cut the stem; then cut the tips and divide them in half, then eliminate the central part, called beard. Put them in a bowl filled with water and lemon juice to prevent them from turning black.

When you have cleaned all the artichokes, cook them in salted water in a pressure cooker for 10 minutes (if you don't have a pressure cooker blanch them for 20 minutes): the artichokes should be tender but not overdone. Meanwhile, cut from a piece of bread (preferably stale), removing the outer crust, 300 g of breadcrumbs and cut it into cubes. Drain the artichokes and place them in a mixer in order to obtain a creamy aspect.

Add salt and pepper, add the breadcrumbs, the grated parmesan and the egg and finally a crushed clove of garlic. Whisk everything until all the ingredients are well mixed.

Transfer the mixture into a bowl and add the chopped parsley. Let the mixture cool and in the meantime, cut the montasio into small cubes, about half a cm. Now make the meatballs: take about 20 g of dough and shape it into a ball with your hands. To shape them easier, wet the palm with water.

With the forefinger, gently press the meatball in the center, forming a small hole in which you will insert a cube of montasio. Turn the dough ball with the two palms, so that the filling is well covered and the meatball is uniform. Once the filling is finished, bread the meatballs by first passing them in the beaten egg and immediately after in the breadcrumbs, which will have to cover them completely. Heat the oil in a large saucepan and when it reaches the necessary temperature (about 180 degrees), fry the meatballs, turning them from time to time, so that they are well browned on all sides. If you don't want to fry the meatballs, you can cook them in the oven at 200° for 25 minutes, until they are golden brown. Drain the meatballs and leave to dry on absorbent paper: serve the artichoke balls with a stringy heart immediately, to better enjoy the montasio filling!

LEMON AND PEPPER OYSTERS

Ingredients
Lemon wedges 3
White pepper q.b.
Oysters 12

Preparation
To make the lemon and pepper oysters, make sure that the oyster shells are closed, then open the oysters, this is a very delicate operation, equip yourself with the special small knife with thin tip, protect your fingers trying to have a firm grip. Hold the oyster firmly with one hand and hold the knife with the other hand and look for the opening (if you want you can ask the fish shop for the oysters to be already drilled for easy opening) insert the blade and cut the muscle that is in the central part. After you have cut it, it will be easier to follow the circumference by fully opening the oyster.

Open the shell in half, being careful not to spill the water from the oysters. The fresher an oyster is, the harder it is to open. If you are not an expert, protect the hand that will hold the oyster with a cloth, to avoid any injuries. Break the ice into the ice crusher and distribute it on a serving plate, put the oysters on the lemon wedges and serve. Each dinner will be seasoned with lemon juice and pepper to taste.

MUSSELS IN WHITE WINE AND CREAM SAUCE

Ingredients for 4 people
Mussels 2 kg
Butter 50 g
Onions 80 g
Garlic 10 g
White wine 400 ml
Lemons 1
Sage q.b.
Rosemary q.b.
Thyme q.b.
Flour 30 g
Parsley 5 g
200 ml liquid fresh cream

Preparation

To prepare the mussels in white wine and cream sauce, start with the aromatic herbs: rinse well and dry. Then remove the thyme and rosemary leaves from the twigs and finely chop them together with the sage. Then chop the parsley, keeping it aside.

Now chop the onion. Grate the lemon peel and collect everything into a small bowl. Squeeze it and get the juice: keep the juice and peel aside.

At this point, devote yourself to cleaning mussels (for more details, see our cooking school: How to clean mussels). Rinse the mussels well under plenty of running water and remove the beard that you will see coming out of the mussel shells. With the help of a small knife, remove all the dirt from the shell and for greater cleaning pass a steel wool on the shell to eliminate the remaining impurities.

Now take a pan with high sides and a non-stick bottom and melt 40 g of butter on very low heat. When it is melted add the garlic and the onion. When the garlic is golden, remove it. Add the white wine and add lemon juice.

Flavor with lemon peel. Add the chopped sage, rosemary and thyme, mixing the ingredients well. Finally add the mussels.

Cover with lid and cook on low heat for 3-4 minutes. When the mussels have opened, using a slotted spoon, transfer them into a bowl and open some by removing the shells.

Reduce the cooking liquid and pour the remaining 10 g of butter that you will melt. Transfer a ladle of the cooking liquid into a large bowl in which you will pour the flour while continuing to whip with the whisk to create a homogeneous mixture without lumps.

Transfer it back into the pan while continuing to mix the ingredients to avoid the formation of lumps: let it thicken on very low heat for 2-3 minutes. Then add the cream, always continuing to whip. Finally pour the mussels back into the pan.

Mix them well with the cooking liquid and let them heat on low heat for 3-4 minutes. Flavor with chopped parsley, mixing it well with the other ingredients and turn off the heat. Finally, add salt and pepper to taste. Serve the mussels now in white wine and cream sauce and enjoy them while still hot.

SHRIMP COCKTAIL

Ingredients for 4 people

Shrimp 16

Iceberg lettuce 60 g

Lemons 4 slices

FOR THE MAYONNAISE

Fresh yolks 1

Sunflower oil 120 g

Filtered lemon juice 15 g

Salt up to q.b.

Black pepper q.b.

FOR THE COCKTAIL SAUCE

Ketchup 45 g

Worcestershire sauce 1 tsp

Tabasco q.b.

Brandy 1 tsp

Preparation

To prepare the shrimp cocktail start with mayonnaise. In the glass of a mixer, pour the egg yolk together with salt, pepper and the filtered lemon juice, then pour the seed oil vey slowly, while operating the immersion blender. After a few moments you will obtaine the mayonnaise of the right creamy consistency.

Move on to the preparation of the cocktail sauce. Pour the mayonnaise into a bowl and add the ketchup, the worcestershire sauce, then the brandy and mix everything. Finally add a few drops of Tabasco, stir again and set aside in a cool place. Switch to cleaning the shrimp: remove all the tails and clean them from the legs and shell, leaving the tail attached. Clean the shrimp by removing the gut which could be bitter. At this point, place 4 tails at a time on a slotted spoon and dip them for about 10 seconds in boiling water, enough time to boil the shrimps and make them curl a little, then drain them on a plate and continue with all the others. Finally cut the iceberg salad into strips and you have everything ready for the composition. In a cocktail glass (or in any other type of glass which is tall and wide), pour a spoonful of cocktail sauce, then add a strip of salad and pour some more sauce. Place 4 shrimps per glass and finally decorate with a slice of lemon. The shrimp cocktail is ready: serve immediately or put it in the fridge for half an hour.

SHRIMP WITH WINE AND LEMON

Ingredients for 4 people

1 kg of shrimps
Parsley
1 clove of garlic
1 glass of white wine
1 lemon juice
Extra virgin olive oil

Preparation

First of all you need to clean the shrimps.
I decided to leave the head and remove the shell but you can choose to remove the head.

Once washed and cleaned, take a pan big enough for all of them to fit, put 3 tablespoons of oil, parsley and garlic. Fry and add the shrimps one at a time in the pan.
Cook for 2 minutes, stir and pour the wine glass. Cook another 2 minutes and then add the lemon juice. Cook for 1 minute more and serve!
Serve with a good white wine!!!

SWORDFISH MEATBALLS WITH LEMON AND OLIVES

Ingredients 4 people
600 g of swordfish
2 potatoes
parmesan
bread crumbs
parsley
milk
organic lemon jam
olives
1 egg
smoked salt
oil
for the sauce
1 pepper
300 g of tomato sauce
1 shallot
oil
salt

Preparation
Wash the potatoes, peel them, cut into slices and steam them with a few grains of smoked salt.
Wash and cook the swordfish in the same way.
Mix both with a potato masher in a bowl and add the Parmesan, parsley and bread crumbs, mix and wet the dough with a little olive oil and a dash of milk and make a firm dough, season with salt.
Take a little bit of the mixture and flatten it on the hand, put in the center a teaspoon of jam and a Taggiasca olive and form the meatballs.
Pass them in beaten egg and in the breadcrumbs, put them in a pan covered with parchment paper and bake at 180 ° for 15 minutes until golden brown, if you want you can fry them more.
Prepare the sauce by roasting the pepper on a flame or on a plate, and then let it cool in a paper bag.

Peel and cut it into small pieces, prepare the sauce by browning the sliced shallot in the oil.

Add the pepper, cook for 10 minutes, season with salt and stir.

You can add some chilli, but not too much so as not to overpower the taste of meatballs.

TUNA MEATBALLS WITH LEMON

Ingredients for 4 people

3 tuna cans of 160 g
2 mashed boiled potatoes
Chopped parsley
Grated lemon peel
1 egg
1 pinch of salt
Bread crumbs
Olive oil
Bread crumbs soaked in milk and squeezed
Finely chopped hazelnuts

Preparation

Drain the tuna well from the preservation oil and place it in a bowl.
Crush it with a fork and add the other ingredients.
Mix everything well and form the meatballs.
Pass them in the breadcrumbs mixed with the chopped hazelnuts and place
the meatballs in a pan covered with greased parchment paper.
Season with a little oil and bake at 200 degrees for about 20 minutes.

CHICKEN, LEMON AND MUSTARD BURGERS

Ingredients for 8 people
For milk sandwiches:
100 g manitoba flour (W 360)
50 g milk
25 g butter
15 g whole egg (3 tablespoons of beaten egg)
8 g milk powder
5 g yeast
4 g granulated sugar
2 g salt
1.5 g barley malt
Sesame and poppy seeds
For mini-burgers:
100 g chicken breast
50 g whole egg (what is left from the sandwiches)
12.5 g butter
7 g mustard beans
1 g lemon juice
1 g parsley
Salt and pepper
Cherry tomatoes
Fresh salad
Mayonnaise
Dijon mustard
Manitoba flour (W 360)
The strength of the flour is measured in W.
A high W indicates a high gluten content.
A low W indicates a flour that needs little water and that rises quickly, but that will give a light and not very thick dough (and a bread). 170W flours are considered (weak): and therefore ideal for biscuits, waffles, breadsticks and desserts. They absorb 50% of their weight in water approximately
180W flour at 260W (medium): French bread, oil rolls, pizza, pasta: they absorb 55% to 65% of their weight in water.

Flour from 280W to 350W (strong) is used for: Pizza, egg pasta, long leavening pastry: babà, brioches. They absorb from 65% to 75% of their weight in water approximately.

Over 350W (special flours): generally made with particular types of wheat, they are used to reinforce "weaker flours", mixing them, or for particular products.

The flour sold in normal shops and supermarkets varies between 150W and 200W, but you can also find Manitoba, with about 400W, to mix it with "normal" flour and obtain the desired strength.

Preparation

Mix the flour with milk, milk powder, egg, baking powder, sugar and malt in a bowl and stir for a long time until the dough is strong. Add the butter and salt and continue to work until completely absorbed.

Form a ball and place it in the bowl, which will be sealed with transparent film. Let it rest for 10 minutes at room temperature, then transfer it into the fridge for 3 hours.

Spend the 3 hours spreading the dough trying to create a thickness of about 1.5 cm and with a round cutter of 3 cm in diameter obtain the micro rolls (you will have about 20), arranging them gradually on a plate covered with parchment paper.

Cover with a sheet of plastic wrap and let rise for half an hour in a warm place, away from streams.

Put in an oven a beaten egg with a small brush then put the poppy and sesame seeds mixed and bake at 180 ° C for 10-15 minutes (check often it takes a moment for them to burn!). Let them cool.

Meanwhile make the hamburgers: chop the meat, add the other ingredients and mix well. The dough remains very soft. Form mini-meatballs 5 mm high and 3 cm wide, with the help of the pastry cutter used for the sandwiches.

Arrange the meatballs on a baking sheet covered with parchment paper and bake at 240 ° C for a few minutes, until they are cooked.

In a small bowl mix the Dijon mustard and mayonnaise to taste (I followed the proportions 1 part of mustard and 3 of mayonnaise).

Cut the sandwiches, stuff with a meatball, the mayonnaise, a slice of cherry tomato and a leaf of salad, fixed with a toothpick and serve.

MARINATED SALMON

Ingredients for 4 people

300 grams of salmon *

2 lemons

1 lime

Salt

Pepper

15 grams of parsley

* for more safety, use frozen or chilled salmon

Material

Food film

Preparation

Cut the salmon into cubes. Squeeze 2 lemons and a lime. Chop the parsley. Stir in a baking dish and add salt and pepper. Stir well and cover the container with the film then let it rest in the refrigerator for 1 hour.

The meal is ready.

SALMON, ROCKET AND ALMOND SALAD

Ingredients

100 g of smoked salmon
30 g of sliced almonds (to toast or already toasted)
A bunch of rocket
8 cherry tomatoes
1 avocado
9 to 12 tablespoons of lemon juice
Extra virgin olive oil
Salt and pepper

Preparation

Toast the almonds in the pan for a few minutes and, in the meantime, cut the salmon into strips and wash the rocket and the tomatoes. Cut the avocado in half, remove the pulp - and cut it into cubes - then slice the tomatoes.

In a bowl combine the vegetables with the fish, the tomatoes and the avocado. Season with extra virgin olive oil, lemon juice, salt and pepper to taste and garnish with toasted almond slices.

Enjoy your meal!

COUSCOUS SALAD

Ingredients for 4 people

200 g of precooked couscous

2 tomatoes

2 spring onions

2 lemons

Fresh mint

Abundant parsley

Oil

Salt

Pepper

Preparation

Place the couscous into a bowl, pour cold water and let it swell for about 20 minutes. Meanwhile, clean the tomatoes trying to eliminate the seeds and cut them into cubes. Finely cut the white part of the onions. Chop abundant parsley and mint leaves. Drain the couscous, press it so that the excess water comes out and put it in a salad bowl. Add the onions, mint, parsley, filtered lemon juice and two tablespoons of oil. Add salt and pepper, stir and refrigerate. Before putting on the table add the diced tomato. Serve with warm Arabic bread.

Enjoy your meal!

CHICKPEA SUMMER SALAD

Ingredients

1 can of chickpeas
150 g of dried tomatoes
150 g of black olives
9 tablespoons of lemon juice
1 stick of tofu
Chives and parsley
Salt and pepper
Extra virgin olive oil

Preparation

Rinse the chickpeas and drain them.

(If you have more time: burn the chickpeas for 5-7 minutes in a pan with a drizzle of oil, chopped onion and a sprinkling of parsley).

Take the dried tomatoes - if you prefer, you can opt for fresh ones - cut them into strips and prepare some diced tofu.

Place the chickpeas, dried tomatoes, tofu cubes and olives in a bowl. Season all with lemon juice, extra virgin olive oil, salt and pepper.

Enjoy your meal!

STRAWBERRY SALAD

Ingredients

100 g strawberries

1 apple

½ stalk of celery

200 g of cheese with herbs

1 head of lettuce

6 walnuts

3 tablespoons of lemon juice

Oil & salt

Preparation

Put the washed and cut salad in a bowl, rinse and cut the strawberries into 4 pieces, slice the apple into cubes, add the walnuts, the chopped celery and the cheese with herbs. Season the salad with lemon juice, a drizzle of extra virgin olive oil, adding salt to taste.

Enjoy your meal!

FRUIT SALAD, LETTUCE, LIME JUICE AND SWEET PROVOLONE

Ingredients
200 g of sweet provolone
4 lettuce hearts
400 g fresh pineapple
4 large strawberries
12 grains of white grapes
150 ml of natural yogurt
6 tablespoons of lemon juice
yogurt q.b.
Sesame seeds for garnish

Preparation
Wash the lettuce hearts and cut them carefully. Arrange the salad in a serving dish. Cut the pineapple into small pieces, the strawberries in slices and the grapes in half, eliminating the seeds.
Put the fruits on a plate with the lettuce and add the diced provolone.
Carefully mix the yogurt with the lemon juice.
Salt the salad to taste, season with the Caribbean-flavored lime sauce and garnish with a sprinkling of sesame seeds.
Enjoy your meal!

ORIENTAL SCENTS SALAD

Ingredients

100 g of curly salad

100 g of valerian

5 cherry tomatoes

1 celery stalk

1 bunch of radishes

300 g of carrots

1 round of 250 g tofu

100 g of bean sprouts

¼ of spring onion

4 tablespoons of extra virgin olive oil

3 tablespoons of lemon juice

2 tablespoons of mixed seeds (flax, pumpkin, sesame)

Apple vinegar and salt

Preparation

Wash the salad carefully, dry it and cut it finely; then, wash, peel and cut the carrots into thin strips. In a bowl, place the bean sprouts, the chopped tomatoes, the chopped onion with a tofu and the seeds. Cut the celery into slices and the radishes: mix everything with the other ingredients and season with extra virgin olive oil, lemon juice, apple vinegar and salt. If you wish, you can add some chives or a pinch of ginger powder. Serve with toasted rye bread.

Enjoy your meal!

SHRIMP AND PINEAPPLE SALAD

Ingredients

500 grams of shrimp

1 whole pineapple

Rocket

Lettuce

Carrots

Valerian

3 tablespoons of lemon juice

4 tablespoons of extra virgin olive oil

Salt

Pepper

Bread croutons

Preparation

Eliminate all the leathery parts and the shrimp filaments and rinse them under running water. After cleaning them, put them into a small pan of boiling salted water and cook for about 3 minutes. Once cooked, drain and let cool. In the meantime, cut the pineapple into large pieces and place it into a bowl together with the cold shrimps. Wash and dry the salad, cut it into small pieces and add it to the bowl where you put the shrimp and pineapple. Do the same with the carrots, cut into julienne strips. Mix everything together, then season with extra virgin olive oil and lemon juice. Add toasted bread croutons to the salad.

Enjoy your meal!

SALAD WITH ARTICHOKES, JERUSALEM ARTICHOKE AND LEMON JUICE

The Jerusalem artichoke is a tuber that resembles the potato in the form and a little the artichoke in the taste. Known as German turnip or Jerusalem artichoke, it reduces cholesterol and stabilizes the concentration of glucose in the blood.

The properties of the artichoke: they promote diuresis, purify, reduce cholesterol, promote digestion and protect the liver.

The rocket with a bitter and firm taste, is a natural source of folic acid, stimulates the appetite and is known to be purifying, detoxifying and very diuretic.

Ingredients
3 artichokes
500 g of Jerusalem artichokes
1 clove of garlic
1 bunch of rocket
1 sprig of parsley
12 tablespoons of lemon juice
Extra virgin olive oil
Salt and pepper

Preparation
Wash the Jerusalem artichokes well, cut them into slices and put them in a solution of water and lemon juice. Even the Jerusalem artichokes like artichokes tend to oxidize.

Wash the artichokes well, remove the tougher outer leaves, cut them in half and remove the internal beard. Slice the artichokes into strips and marinate them in a bowl with water, lemon juice, salt and pepper.

Pour a little extra virgin olive oil and the poached garlic clove in a pan. Add the Jerusalem artichoke and season to taste. Put some white wine, add a sprinkling of parsley and cook for about 20 minutes, adding a little water.

Wash the rocket and place it on the plate. Combine the marinating of artichokes, the Jerusalem artichokes
and season w th lemon juice and extra virgin olive oil.
Enjoy your meal!

POTATO SALAD WITH AROMATIC HERBS AND CITRUS JUICE

Ingredients
6 new potatoes
1 shallot
2 celery hearts
Parsley
Basil
Chives
4 tablespoons of lemon juice
1 tablespoon of extra virgin olive oil
For the juice
1 orange
1 pink grapefruit
1 teaspoon of lemon juice
What you need: pot

Preparation
Wash the potatoes very carefully and put them together with the peel in a pan with plenty of cold water. Once it reaches boiling, cook for about 20 minutes.
Meanwhile wash and clean the celery, then cut into small pieces of about half a centimeter. Clean the shallot and chop it. Wash the parsley and the basil. When the potatoes have cooled, peel them. Then prepare an emulsion with extra virgin olive oil, lemon juice and a pinch of salt. Once cooled, cut the potatoes into pieces, add celery, shallots and season with the oil and lemon emulsion. Finally sprinkle with chopped parsley and a few basil leaves. Accompany all with a fresh citrus juice made of an orange, a grapefruit and lemon juice.
Enjoy your meal!

LIGHT SALAD WITH SALMON

Ingredients

5 slices of smoked salmon

5 radishes

1 bunch of mixed salad

10 fresh tomatoes

1/2 green pepper

Half red tropea onion

10 black olives without stones

2 tablespoons of lemon juice equal to half a lemon

Preparation

Wash all the vegetables well. Then add the radishes cut into very thin slices in a large bowl and add the salad leaves, the chopped tomatoes into four equal parts, the onion and green pepper cut into thin strips. Add the lemon juice. Cut the salmon into small pieces and add to the salad and stir.

Enjoy your meal!

DRESSING

BECHAMEL SAUCE AT THE MAÎTRE D'HÔTEL

Ingredients for 4 people
Bechamel
40 g of butter
1 lemon
1 tablespoon of chopped parsley

Preparation
Make the bechamel sauce by using the doses of the basic recipe. When it is ready dilute it with 4-5 tablespoons of hot water, mixing well. Bring it to a light boil, then add the strained lemon juice and the chopped parsley. Mix the mixture, remove it and stir in the butter.
Enjoy your meal!

COMPOUND BUTTER ALLA MUGNAIA

Ingredients

100 g of butter

Lemon

Salt

Pepper

Preparation

Put the butter in a small pan and let it melt on low heat. As soon as it is completely melted, add two tablespoons of filtered lemon juice to the strainer, a pinch of salt and one of pepper.

Enjoy your meal!

MARINADE IN VINEGAR

Ingredients

1 glass of white vinegar

1 lemon

1 glass of oil

Parsley

Rosemary

Oregano

Salt

Pepper

Preparation

Mix the vinegar with oil and lemon juice, then pour it into a large bowl. Add a tablespoon of rosemary needles and one or two of chopped parsley, a pinch of oregano, salt and pepper. Put the fish and let it cook for two hours before eating it.

Enjoy your meal!

FIRST COURSES

PENNE WITH ASPARAGUS AND LEMON PESTO

Ingredients
500 g of penne
1 bunch of asparagus
50 g of parmesan cheese
50 g of pine nuts
3 tablespoons of lemon juice
Extra virgin olive oil
1 garlic clove
Parsley
Salt and pepper

Preparation
Wash the asparagus and boil in salted water for about 15-20 minutes, until they become tender. Drain well, cut the tips (which you will put aside) and dice the stems. In a mixer, prepare the pesto by adding the diced asparagus with Parmesan, garlic clove, pine nuts, lemon juice, parsley, salt and pepper. Reduce all the ingredients to a cream and slowly add the extra virgin olive oil.
Cook the pasta, drain and season with the freshly prepared pesto, adding the asparagus heads and a generous sprinkling of Parmesan.
Enjoy your meal!

TAGLIATELLE BOTTARGA, CLAMS AND LEMON

Ingredients

400 g Tagliatelle

1 kg of clams

40 g of Bottarga

20 ml of lemon juice

1 clove of garlic

1 sprig of parsley

Salt and Pepper to taste

Extra virgin olive oil q.b.

Preparation

Wash the clams: check that they do not contain sand, beat them one by one on a cutting board on the opening: if dark sand comes out it means that the clam has to be thrown away. Eliminate also those with a broken shell. Once this selection has been made, place the clams in a colander resting on a bowl and rinse them several times under running water, finishing only when there is no more sand in the bowl.

Take a large pan and pour a little oil, a crushed clove of garlic, browning it for a few moments.

Drain the clams well and put them into the pan covering with a lid heating on a flame high enough so that the valves open from heat. When all the clams open, turn off the heat.

At this point, drain the clams and keep the formed cooking liquid. Peel half of the clams and pour them into a large pan with the cooking liquid, adding the lemon juice. Boil the water in a large pot, add salt and add the noodles for a few minutes. In the meantime, chop the bottarga and chop the parsley pepper to taste.

Drain the tagliatelle dressing with the clam, lemon sauce, chopped bottarga and parsley, and serve hot.

Enjoy your meal!

LEMON RICE WITH VEGETABLES

Ingredients
320 grams of rice
1 shallot
½ onion
4 carrots
2 zucchini
2 celery
50 ml of lemon juice
Salt to taste
15 ml of extra virgin olive oil
White wine q.b.
What you need: pot, pan

Preparation
Wash and clean the carrots, zucchini and celery well, keeping the latter's leaves aside. Put all the vegetables in a saucepan covering with plenty of cold water, then bring to boil and let simmer.

Meanwhile, chop the shallots and the onion and brown them in a pan with 10 ml of oil. Add the rice, toast it for 1 minute and add a little white wine.

Salt the vegetable broth and occasionally add it to the rice, stirring constantly.

When cookec, add the lemon juice and 5 ml of oil and let it stir for a few minutes. Wash some celery leaves. Add carrots and celery for decoration.

Enjoy your meal!

PAPPARDELLE WITH VEGETABLES

Ingredients for 4 people

400 gr of pappardelle

2 artichokes

2 zucchini

1 eggplant

10 taggiasche olives

Lemon juice 12 tablespoons

Chives q.b.

1 shallot

Curcuma q.b.

Salt and Pepper to taste.

Preparation

Clean the artichokes and cut them into wedges, then dip them in a bowl with water and lemon juice (12 tablespoons).

Cut the shallot, let it simmer a little with EVO (Extra Virgin Olive Oil) and add the artichokes. Sauté for a few minutes in the pan, and then add a glass of water.

Cut the courgettes and the eggplant into cubes which you will then add to the artichokes being cooked. Season with salt, pepper and a little turmeric to taste. Add the chives to the vegetables.

Separately, cook the pappardelle. When they reach cooking, drain and sauté in a pan with the vegetables.

Serve sprinkling with grana or pecorino. The hot pepper on this dish is ideal for those who can afford it.

Enjoy your meal!

BAVETTE WITH LEMON AND SAUSAGE

Ingredients for 4 people

400 g bavette
200 g of sausage
3 tablespoons of lemon juice
Parsley
Extra virgin olive oil

Preparation

Pour a drizzle of oil in a pan, add the lemon juice, the sausage and the chopped parsley. Cook for a few minutes, the time required for all the flavors of the ingredients to mix. Meanwhile cook the bavette and at the end of the cooking add them to the previously prepared dressing.

Finish the preparation by adding a sprig of parsley.

Enjoy your meal!

BARLEY AND MELON SOUP

Ingredients for 4 people
250 g of pearl barley
1 heart of green celery with leaves
1 lemon
40 g of almonds with the peel
1 dozen Taggiasche olives
1 dozen green olives
1/2 melon
1 clove of garlic
2 sprigs of thyme
Extra virgin olive oil
Black pepper
Salt

Preparation
Rinse and cook the barley in salted water with the crushed garlic clove and the sprigs of thyme tied so that they can be tied together for about 40 minutes, eliminating the foam that forms on the surface. Drain it, remove the garlic and the thyme and let it cool.

Remove the hazelnut from the olives and add it to the barley. Remove the celery leaves, wash them, dry them and blend them with almonds, filtered juice of half a lemon, 5-6 tablespoons of oil, a pinch of salt and a generous grinding of pepper. Season the barley and stir.

Take strips of celery with a potato peeler and place them in cold water. Cut the others into cubes and add them to the barley. Clean the melon, take 8 balls with the round scoop and cut them into slices. Puree the pulp with salt pepper and oil.

Arrange the barley salad in four pastry rings placed in the center of four soup plates, cover it with the melon slices and the drained celery strips, then dry and pour around the melon soup. Gently remove the pastry rings, complete with another round of pepper and serve.

Enjoy your meal!

CALAMARI, CAPERS AND LEMON

Ingredients for 4 people

300 g calamarata

2 clean squids

1 handful of salted capers

1 shallot

1 untreated lemon

A few sprigs of thyme

1/2 glass of white wine

Preparation

Clean the squid and cut it into very thin rings. Fry the shallot in the pan. Put the squid and cook on high heat, then blend with the wine and let it dry. Put the capers that you previously washed well and cook with a tablespoon of water. While cooking the Calamarata, cut the lemon peel into long, thin strips, taking care to remove the white part. Drain the pasta and stir in a hot flame for a few moments, then add the lemon and the olive oil. Serve hot, perfuming with fresh thyme.

Enjoy your meal!

EGG, LEMON, ROSEMARY AND PINK PEPPER TAGLIATELLE

Ingredients for 3 people

250 g of Tagliatelle with egg
1 lemon
1 sprig of rosemary
100 ml fresh cream for cooking
Pink pepper
Salt

Preparation

Grate some lemon peel. Chop the rosemary and add it to the pan. Add the fresh cream, salt and cook for about a minute, then crumble a few grains of pink pepper to give a little sparkle but do not overdo it.

Cook the egg noodles in abundant salted water, drain and add them to the sauce. Let them season for a few seconds and serve with lemon zest, fresh rosemary and a glass of dry white wine.

Enjoy your meal!

SPAGHETTI WITH OLIVES, ANCHOVIES, LEMON

Ingredients for 4 people
360 g of spaghetti alla chitarra
8 anchovy fillets in oil
8 tablespoons of black olives without stones
Parsley to taste
¼ clove of garlic
4 tablespoons of stale bread without crust
Grated peel of half a lemon
Extra virgin olive oil

Introduction
Olives, anchovies, parsley and the refreshing touch of grated lemon peel are all you need. Easy to find ingredients, at a reduced cost, which we usually all have in the pantry. With the stale bread, crumbled coarsely and browned in a pan with a little oil, you will complete the dish with a toasted note and an unexpected crunchiness.

Preparation
Cook the pasta in abundant salted water. Meanwhile crumble the bread crumbs (you can use a blender to speed up the operation) and brown it in a pan with two tablespoons of extra virgin olive oil. Blend the anchovies together with the olives, garlic and lemon zest, finishing with the oil until you get a fairly creamy sauce. Add the chopped parsley and mix. Drain the pasta al dente and add the crunchy crumb.
Enjoy your meal!

TOMATO AND LEMON RISOTTO

Ingredients for 4 people
8 cherry tomatoes
8 peeled tomatoes
4 dried tomatoes
240 g of rice
White wine
Butter
Oil
Grated lemon peel
1 handful of parmesan cheese
1 pinch of sweet paprika
1 pinch of strong paprika
1 shallot

Preparation
Dip the dried tomatoes in warm water for an hour. Dip the fresh tomatoes in the boiling water, peel them, cut them and remove the seeds. Add the peeled and cut tomatoes. Pour in lightly browned garlic flavored oil and let it warm up for 5 minutes. Add the dried tomatoes and blend.

Prepare a small shallot stew. Toast the rice for three minutes. Add white wine and blend, add the shallot cream. Cook with salted water. Add the tomato, a small piece of butter, a tablespoon of oil and stir off the heat with a handful of Parmesan, a pinch of sweet paprika and a pinch of spice. Put on the plate and grate some lemon on top.

Enjoy your meal!

SPICY LEMON LINGUINE

Ingredients for 6 people

500 g of linguine
10 tablespoons of oil
4 dried peppers
4 untreated lemons
Salt
Pepper

Preparation

Heat the water for cooking the pasta. In the meantime, heat two tablespoons of oil in a pan, add the peppers and, stirring them occasionally, let them soften for about 10 minutes and then remove them, they will have already transferred the fragrance to the oil.

Cook the linguine in salted water for 7 or 8 minutes. Pass them in the oil pan with chilli pepper, add the grated peel of two lemons and six tablespoons of their juice the strainer, stir them for a few seconds, adding a tablespoon of cooking water if necessary.

Transfer the linguine to the serving dish, season with freshly ground pepper and serve immediately. Garnish with wedges of the remaining lemons.

Enjoy your meal!

LEMON MEATBALLS IN BROTH

Ingredients for 4 people

1 l of meat broth

100 g of butter

3 eggs

40 g of grated cheese

50 g of bread crumbs

2 tablespoons of lemon juice

Salt

Pepper

Preparation

Melt the butter in a pan, then add the egg yolks and bread crumbs, stirring quickly. Add salt and pepper. Mix the mixture with the whipped egg whites until stiff. Let it rest for an hour. Make lots of balls as big as nuts. Cook them in the broth for a few minutes. Serve with cheese.

Enjoy your meal!

LEMON AND BASIL RISOTTO

Ingredients for 4 people

320 g of rice
1 lemon
1 glass of dry white wine
1 l of vegetable broth
1/2 onion
1 shallot
10 fresh basil leaves
Butter
3 tablespoons of oil
Salt
Pepper

Preparation

In a saucepan, heat two tablespoons of oil, finely chop the onion and shallot, and when they are transparent, add the rice. Jumble up. After a minute put some wine and wait for it to evaporate. Add salt. Cook the risotto by pouring a ladle of hot broth at a time. Five minutes after cooking, add a teaspoon of grated lemon peel. When the rice is ready, whisk it with a little butter and a drizzle of oil, the lemon juice, a pinch of pepper and the chopped basil. Stir, let stand a minute and then serve.

Enjoy your meal!

LINGUINE WITH SWORDFISH AND LEMON

Ingredients

A nice slice of fresh swordfish

1 lemon

5 grams of butter

A drizzle of extra virgin olive oil

Salt and pepper to taste

Preparation

Put a pot of water on fire and start cleaning the fish. Swordfish does not contain scales and is therefore easy to prepare. You just have to get rid of the skin and the central bone. To make it easier, use a sharp knife. Remove the peel, and cut four pieces of clean meat. As soon as the water for the pasta has reached the boiling point, add a handful of salt and then the linguine (or pasta you have chosen to cook). You probably haven't finished cleaning the fish yet, or, if you've been quick, you can move on to the next step.
Cut the fish into cubes. Wash the lemon and grate the peel.
Now put the butter and a drizzle of extra-virgin olive oil in a ladle. Place the ladle over the pot in which you are cooking the pasta, for a few seconds. The heat will melt the butter together with the oil. Keep the liquid aside.

Take a skewer and pour the ladle of oil and butter, the pieces of swordfish, mint, lemon zest (leave aside a little to garnish the dishes), the juice of half a lemon and a pinch of salt and pepper. Mix. The stove must be switched off.

At this point, the pasta will be almost ready. Drain it and pour it into the wok, along with the one you prepared earlier. Light the fire and cook for no more than two minutes. After the first minute, add the juice of the other lemon half. And mix again. Turn off the heat and start serving.

Create a nest with your long pasta.
If you have chosen to cook long pasta, such as spaghetti or linguine, use this ploy to serve. Take a fork and a kitchen ladle. You can use the one where you melted the butter. It will be fine. Rotate the linguine in the ladle and place it in a shallow dish. Advisable in the center. Beautify with the lemon peel you set aside earlier.
The dish is ready.

PASTA WITH GORGONZOLA GINGER PUMPKIN

Ingredients for 4 people
About 300 grams of red pumpkin
A slice of ginger 1 cm thick
Rind of half grated lemon
30 grams of sweet gorgonzola
Salt and pepper to taste

Preparation
The preparation of today's fast first course is simple, quick and effective.
 Light the fire on the stove. The water will slowly start to warm up. We begin to clean the red pumpkin depriving it of seeds and peel. I suggest you use a sharp knife so you don't have to use too much force in this operation. Cut into thick slices.
Ginger is also sliced and blended. Only one slice will suffice, since the aroma of this spice is quite strong.
Certainly, once the pumpkin and ginger have been cleaned, the water will have reached the ideal temperature to add salt and immediately afterwards dip the pumpkin slices you have made in addition to the ginger one in the pot. Next, add enough pasta to the pot.

RICE WITH ARTICHOKES AND SWORDFISH

Ingredients for 3 people

200 g of rice
100 g of artichoke stalks
70 g of swordfish
A fresh spring onion
Extra virgin olive oil
Salt and pepper
Half a glass of white wine
Half a lemon

Preparation

Use half of the onion needed for rice. Put the rest in a saucepan together with the leathery part you removed from the stems, any outer leaves of the artichoke included. Add a piece of lemon peel.

Use a rather large pan in which you will pour a little extra virgin olive oil. Light the stove on low heat and pour the sliced spring onion. Leave to brown for a few seconds, adding very little water to prevent the onion from burning. As soon as the onion is golden, pour the artichoke stalks, cut into cubes, into a pan, and let them brown for a minute. After that add the rice. Toast it for a minute. It will be at this time that you will have to add salt.

Blend everything with white wine. Half a glass will suffice. As soon as the wine has evaporated, pour the vegetable broth that you have created with the artichoke stem scraps, the spring onion and the lemon rind into the pot. Continue cooking the risotto, adding the broth, until it is perfect.

When cooked, add the swordfish cut into pieces. Let it cook for another minute, the time to cook the pieces of swordfish and melt their flavor by putting it on the plate. Season with salt and pepper. So serve up. Rice with artichokes and swordfish is at its best, if accompanied by a rain of grated lemon peel. This ingredient will enhance the flavor of the fish, which will be accompanied by the sweet aftertaste of the artichoke.

PENNE WITH CITRUS PESTO

Ingredients

Five black olives without kernels

A sprig of rosemary

The rind of a small lemon

The peel of half an orange

Extra virgin olive oil

3 walnut kernels

Salt as needed

Preparation

Fill a pot with water, enough to cook the amount of pasta you want. Put it on the stove and turn it on.

While waiting for the water to boil, arrange the ingredients on your work surface.

Rinse both the orange and the lemon well. You must be sure that the rind is perfectly clean, because it will be the part that you will have to use for the preparation of the recipe. Clean the walnuts and rinse the rosemary too. When the water boils put the pasta you have chosen to use.

Now peel the orange and lemon with a potato peeler. I suggest you use this tool to avoid using the whitish part of the peel in the recipe, which has a rather bitter taste. In the rind, on the other hand, essential oils are contained. The ones that give the dish a delicious aroma and taste. Set aside a lemon zest and an orange zest for the dish decoration. At this point, take the hand blender. In the glass, add extra virgin olive oil, the 3 walnut kernels, the orange and lemon peel and the rosemary leaves, without the stem. Also add 2 ladles of pasta cooking water. It will make the citrus pesto easier to blend. Mix all the ingredients until you get a smooth and homogeneous sauce.

As soon as the pasta is cooked, you just need to drain it and put it back in the pot. The next step? Add the citrus pesto to the pasta. Nothing could be easier. Give a nice stir, to mix everything. Serve your citrus pesto with a shower of orange and lemon zest, cut very thin (you can also grate veiling). The ones you kept aside during the preparation of the recipe. In this way, the taste of the recipe is a little more delicate.

Finally, bring it to the table.

Are you enjoying this book? I would be happy if you could leave a short review on Amazon, it means a lot to me! Thank you!

PASTA WITH CRISPY AUBERGINES AND LEMON PEEL

Ingredients

1 eggplant of about 150 g

1 lemon

30 g of ricotta cheese

Extra virgin olive oil

Salt and pepper to taste

Preparation

Put a saucepan with enough water to cook the pasta.

Wash the aubergines well before cutting them into small cubes.

Pour a drizzle of extra virgin olive oil in a non-stick pan. As soon as it is hot, add the eggplant cubes and a pinch of salt. Cook well until they are crispy. Take the right amount of pasta and set it aside, for it to be ready to be put in the pot as soon as the water has boiled.

Separately, grate the rind of a fresh lemon. Immediately after the ricotta cheese.

One last thing is still missing. You need some chopped pistachio or other dried fruit. You can use the one you consider most appropriate, or at least, the one you have in the pantry.

Almonds, walnuts, cashews or pistachios will make your first meal delicious. You only need 4 or 5 pistachios (if you use nuts, even 1/2 walnut). Shell the dried fruit and place it in a clean napkin. Crush them roughly with a meat mallet.

Now all the ingredients should be ready.

Perfectly cooked pasta, crunchy aubergine cubes. On the side you have grated lemon rind and coarsely chopped nuts. All you have to do is unite everything. Drain the pasta, pour it back into the pan where you cooked it. Proceed by adding oil and fried aubergines, sprinkle with rind of lemon peel and crumbled dried fruit. Mix everything, taking care to leave aside some lemon zest and grains. You will need them to color the dish before bringing it to the table. The yellow of the lemon and the green of the pistachio give your first appearance appetizing.

LINGUINE WITH DRIED TOMATO PESTO AND LEMON PEEL

Ingredients for 2 people

1 ripe lemon

4 dried tomatoes (2 per person)

40 g of salted ricotta (or ricotta cheese)

Extra virgin olive oil

Half a clove of aglione (if you don't have the aglione use half a clove of garlic)

Pasta cooking water

Preparation

Start preparing the dish by boiling enough water to cook about 200 grams of pasta. A quantity sufficient for 2 people.

Meanwhile, arrange all the ingredients on your work plan. Having everything at your fingertips will help you speed up your preparation time and keep you from looking in the pantry.

Wash the lemon well and remove the zest with the help of a potato peeler.

As soon as the water reaches the boiling point, add 4 dried tomatoes to the pan. In this way you will make them rehydrate, making them softer. Blanch for about 3 minutes.

Remove the dried tomatoes, add the salt to the pan and then put the pasta. Peel the garlic and place it in the glass of the immersion blender together with extra virgin olive oil, the dried tomatoes that you have blanched and the lemon rind.

Cover everything with cooking water and mix. Blend until the mixture is soft and smooth.

SECOND COURSES

RECIPES WITH LEMONS

From soufflé to tart. From mousse to meatballs. Passing by risotto and chicken. Up to the famous doc liqueur, limoncello. Lemons are the most used citrus in the kitchen, for the scent they give us, for their ability to give a particular flavor to each dish, for the extraordinary properties they contain. Lemons, including the white part, prevent any type of cardiovascular disease. Furthermore lemons are rich in vitamin C, have few calories and a low glycemic index.

MACKEREL WITH LEMON AND CHILLI PEPPER

Ingredients for 4 people
8 mackerels of about 150 g each
2 lemons
2 apples
1 celery stalk
Lettuce
Fresh chilli
Salt
Pepper

Preparation
Remove the inner part of the mackerel, dry them and with the help of a knife open them in half following the line of the belly. With the scissors clean and remove the bones or any remaining scales.
Cut the lemons in slices and remove the peel, remove the seeds from the chili pepper, then chop them. Inside the fish add salt, pepper, chilli pepper and lemon slices.
Tie the fish with string, then grill them by turning them on both sides.
Finally prepare a salad with celery, apple and lettuce and season with a citronette (made with oil, lemon and salt).
Enjoy your meal!

ESCALOPES WITH LEMON

Ingredients for 4 people
800 g of thinly sliced veal breast
1 lemon
1 clove of garlic
 Flour
Extra virgin olive oil
1 knob of butter
Salt
Pepper
Parsley

Preparation
Start by beating the slices of veal, placed between two sheets of parchment paper, using a meat tenderizer. Alternatively you can ask the butcher to do it for you. Sprinkle flour on the both sides of the slices and brown them on a high heat, evenly, in a saucepan with the garlic, oil and butter.

Grate the thin lemon rind you will keep aside. Squeeze and strain the lemon juice, which you will pour over the escalopes. Season with salt and pepper, then lower the heat and continue cooking for a few minutes.

Serve the lemon escalopes with a sprinkling of freshly ground pepper, grated rind and parsley to taste.

Enjoy your meal!

BAKED LEMON CHICKEN

Ingredients for 4 people
1 chicken of 1 kg and about 200 grams
2 lemons
40 g of butter
1 clove of garlic
1 sprig of parsley
Oil
Salt
Black pepper

Preparation
Begin by massaging the meat with a lemon half on the outer part, add three to four slices of lemon, half butter and a clove of garlic. In a baking dish, heat two tablespoons of oil with the remaining butter, place the chicken on top, salt and pepper, transfer into a hot pan on a hot oven at 180 ° and cook for 1 hour and 15 minutes.

When it is half-cooked, sprinkle with the juice of the remaining lemon, by squeezing. When cooked, take out the chicken and place it on a cutting board. Cut the back and the breast into four parts, remove the wings and the thighs and place everything in the pan, or on a serving plate. Sprinkle with the finely chopped parsley and immediately serve the baked lemon chicken, accompanied with fried or roasted potatoes to taste.

Enjoy your meal!

STRIPED CHICKEN WITH LEMON, HONEY AND ROSEMARY

Ingredients for 4 people

500 g of chicken breast
1/2 glass of dry white wine
Flour to taste
3-4 star anise berries
3 cm of grated ginger
Fresh rosemary
1 tablespoon of delicate fluid honey
1 shallot
Extra virgin olive oil
1 knob of butter
Salt
Pepper

Preparation

Cut the chicken breast into slices of about 1 cm on each side and then into strips. Pass them repeatedly in a dish where you have collected the flour.
Chop the shallots and sauté in a pan with the oil and butter. When it is golden, add the chicken and brown it on a high heat, stirring frequently. Pour the white wine and let the alcohol evaporate.
Add the rind and filtered lemon juice, grated ginger, honey, rosemary and anise.
Enjoy your meal!

CHICKEN WITH GRAPES

Ingredients for 4 people

1 kg of chicken
150 g of grapes
20 g of butter
2 shallots
1 lemon
2 sprig of rosemary
1/2 glass of dry white wine
Oil
Salt
Pepper

Preparation

Squeeze the lemon, strain the juice and use it to carefully wet the chicken. In a saucepan, which can go into the oven, heat a knob of butter with a little oil and add the meat.

Let it brown on high heat turning it from time to time. Pour the white wine, let the alcohol evaporate and add rosemary, salt and pepper. Transfer everything into a pre-heated oven at 180 ° and cook, stirring occasionally, for about 40 minutes.

In a pan, melt the remaining butter and season the chopped shallots, add the grapes, washed and dried. Cook on low heat for a few minutes, stirring occasionally.

When ready to serve, place the chicken in a large serving dish, garnish with the grape mixture and pour the cooking sauce over it.

Enjoy your meal!

LEMON ESCALOPES WITH TURKEY

Ingredients for 4 people
500 g of sliced turkey breast
Flour
2 dl of dry white wine
1 juicy lemon
1 tablespoon of chopped marjoram
1 tablespoon chopped parsley
Extra virgin olive oil
1 knob of butter
Salt

Preparation
Divide the turkey into smaller slices of about 3 fingers per side and flour them. In a non-stick pan heat the butter with a few tablespoons of oil and brown the escalopes 3-4 minutes on each side until they are golden on both sides.
Set them aside while cleaning the frying pan with absorbent kitchen paper.
Put the escalopes in the pan again and place it on the fire, pour in the wine and the lemon juice. Add salt and continue cooking on medium heat for a few minutes, until the bottom of it is partially absorbed becoming thicker. Sprinkle with chopped herbs, stir the escalopes in the sauce to flavor and remove from the heat. Serve immediately.
Enjoy your meal!

CHICKEN WITH LEMON

Ingredients for 4 people
1 chicken (about 1 kg and 200 g)
2 untreated lemons
30 g of butter
1 clove of garlic
1 sprig of parsley
Extra virgin olive oil
Salt
Pepper

Preparation
Wash the chicken carefully and dry it with kitchen paper. Season and salt the chicken in the inner part and rub the outer one with a lemon half. Cut the other half of the lemon into thin slices and arrange them in the abdominal cavity with the whole clove of garlic with the peel and 15 grams of butter. Tie the chicken with a few strings of kitchen string to keep it in shape during cooking.

Place 2 tablespoons of oil in a baking pan covered with baking paper, add the remaining butter, add the chicken, add salt and pepper and bake in a preheated oven at 180 ° for an hour and 15 minutes. Halfway through cooking, place all the juice of the second lemon on the meat. Once cooked transfer the chicken to a cutting board and, using the carving scissors, divide the back and the breast into four pieces, remove the wings and the thighs and place everything on the serving dish, recomposing the chicken as if it were whole. Sprinkle with finely chopped parsley and serve the lemon chicken on the table, accompanied, as desired, with fried or roasted potatoes.

Enjoy your meal!

BAKED SEA BASS WITH LEMON, THYME AND OLIVES

Ingredients for 4 people

4 very large sea bass fillets
2 lemons
50 g of black olives
Fresh thyme
300 g of potatoes
Plenty of parchment paper
Kitchen string

Preparation

Cut the potatoes into thin slices and cook for 5 minutes in salted water.

Clean the sea bass, then season it with oil, salt, pepper and fresh thyme.

Chop the black olives and cut the lemons into 6 slices and put them on the fillets.

Prepare a sheet of parchment paper that is 3 times larger than the fillet of the sea bass. Lay it out on a table and create two folds of 1/3 and 2/3. Spread the fillet, cover with the sliced potatoes and sprinkle with salt. Cover the sides with two edges of parchment paper. Turn the package over. Fold the two long open sides towards the center, making a flap, make two holes on the lapel so that you can pass the string and close them with a bow. Repeat everything for each sea bass fillet.

Bake in a preheated oven at 180 ° C, with a fan, for about 20 minutes. Take it out of the oven and serve it on a plate with all the foil.

For the lazy, the option always remains valid, aluminum foil, roll and go. In any case ... Buon Appetito!

SWORD CARPACCIO WITH AUBERGINE CAVIAR

Ingredients for 6 people

500 g of thin sliced swordfish

2 lemons

Oil

Oregano

Salt

Pepper

For the eggplant caviar

3 eggplants

1 lemon

2 tomatoes

1 clove of garlic

Parsley

Oil

Salt

Preparation

In a bowl, prepare a marinade with lemon juice, oil, oregano, salt and pepper. Place the slices of swordfish, cover with plastic wrap and leave to flavor for a few hours in the fridge. When ready to serve, drain and place them on the serving dish, leaving the center empty. Strain the marinade and pour it over the fish.

Cut the aubergines into slices. Blanch them for four minutes. Take them with the spatula, place them on a cloth and let them cool. Pass them through the vegetable cutter to obtain a puree. Put the lemon juice, garlic, parsley and chopped tomatoes, oil and salt. Arrange the "caviar" in the center of the plate and serve.

Enjoy your meal!

CARPACCIO MARINATED WITH RADICCHIO

Ingredients for 3 people

400 g of veal carpaccio
1/2 lemon
2 sprigs of thyme
1 sprig of rosemary
30 g of parmesan cheese
2 small heads of radicchio
Extra virgin olive oil
Salt

Preparation

Spread the slices of meat on a baking sheet lined with baking paper, season with a pinch of salt, three tablespoons of oil, the juice of half a lemon and the chopped thyme and rosemary leaves.

Cook the meat for 10 minutes and in the meantime peel and cut the radicchio into thin strips, wash and dry it.

Heat the oven grill, place the pan about 20 centimeters from the bottom and cook the meat for 3-4 minutes. Serve it warm with the radicchio seasoned with oil and salt and sprinkled with parmesan cut into flakes.

Enjoy your meal!

STURGEON WITH OIL AND LEMON

Ingredients for 4 people

1 sturgeon (about 1 kg and 200 g)

1 lemon

1 tablespoon chopped parsley

Oil

Salt and pepper

For the court-bouillon:

2 1/2 liters of water

2 dl of dry white wine

2 baby carrots

1 spring onion

1 celery stalk

4 peppercorns

Salt

Preparation

Prepare the court-bouillon: pour the water and the wine into a saucepan, add the carrots, the onion, the celery stalk, the peppercorns and a pinch of salt, simmer for 45 minutes, remove and let cool. Dip the sturgeon in the cold court-bouillon, place on the stove, bring to a light boil, then simmer for 15 minutes, remove and let the sturgeon cool in its cooking broth. Drain it, cut it into four slices, place them on a serving dish. In a bowl mix four tablespoons of oil with two lemon juice, parsley, a pinch of salt and one of pepper. Put the preparation on the sturgeon steaks and after 10 minutes serve on the table. With the stretched court-bouillon you can make an excellent risotto.

Enjoy your meal!

SAN PIETRO FILLETS BOILED IN OIL AND LEMON

Ingredients for 4 people
1 kg and 500 g of San Pietro
Oil
Lemon
Salt

For the court-bouillon
5 l of water
1/2 glass of dry white wine
1 spring onion
1 baby carrot
A celery
4 grains of black pepper
Salt

San Pietro fish: salt water fish, belonging to the Zeidae family.

Preparation
Prepare the court-bouillon: pour the ingredients indicated in a casserole and bring to a light boil, dip the fish and cook for about 30 minutes. Drain it, gently remove the skin and cut it into four pieces. In a bowl, mix four tablespoons of oil with two lemon juice and a pinch of salt. Transfer the fillets onto the serving dish. Serve.

SEA BASS WITH LEMON AND PARSLEY SAUCE

Ingredients for 4 people

1 sea bass of 1 kg and 200 g

350 g of fish stock

150 g of parsley leaves

50 g of oil

4 lemons

Corn flour

Whole grain salt

Lemon grass

Preparation

Cut the lemons into slices about 1/2 inch thick and arrange them on a plate alternating with layers of whole coarse salt. Let it sit for a day. Blanch the parsley, cool it in ice water, drain and blend it with the oil, and a pinch of cornstarch. Pass the mixture through a sieve. Slice the sea bass. Arrange the lemon slices on the bottom of a baking dish and sprinkle them with some lemon grass leaves. Put the sea bass on the lemon slices and place in a hot oven at 180 ° and cook for about ten minutes. Transfer it onto the serving dish and serve with the parsley sauce aside. Sprinckle with chopped chives and parsley and mix well to blend the aromas.

Enjoy your meal!

VEAL SLICES WITH LEMON JUICE AND CAPERS

Ingredients for 6 people

1 kg of magatello
1/2 glass of oil
4 lemons
100 g of capers
1 carrot
1 onion
1 celery stalk
Salt

Preparation

Boil the water in a saucepan with celery, carrot, onion and boil for 2 hours tied with white kitchen string. Let the meat cool in its broth, untie it, cut it into very thin slices, place them onto the serving dish and sprinkle them with washed and unsalted capers.

In a bowl, mix the oil with the lemon juice, add salt and pour over the meat. Leave to soak for half an hour and serve.

Enjoy your meal!

Magatello: precious part of the bovine.

ANCHOVIES WITH CITRUS FRUITS

Ingredients for 4 people

600 g of small boned anchovies

4 oranges

4 lemons

1 bunch of parsley

Chili pepper

Oil

Salt

Pepper

Preparation

Wash the anchovies, dry them and put them in a bowl in a single layer, sprinkle them with the juice of three lemons and let them marinate for about an hour so that the citrus juice "cook" them.

After this time, drain them very well, eliminating all the dark liquid that has formed. Arrange them radially in a serving dish.

Prepare the sauce: in a bowl mix the juice of three oranges with oil, salt, pepper and chilli, then pour it on the anchovies. Cut three slices of orange and lemon from the remaining ones, peel them, make small triangles from each slice and place them on the anchovies, then sprinkle them with finely chopped parsley, let them rest for a few minutes and serve.

Enjoy your meal!

MILANESE-STYLE VEAL SHANKS

Ingredients for 4 people

 4 veal shanks

80 g of butter

1/2 glass of dry white wine

2 tablespoons of tomato paste

1/2 onion

1 carrot

1 celery stalk

Flour

Salt

Pepper

For the "GREMATA"

1/2 lemon peel

Parsley

For the risotto

350 g of rice

20 g of beef marrow

1 l and 1/2 of meat broth

1 small onion

1 sachet of saffron

80 g of grated cheese

80 g of butter

Salt

Preparation

In a saucepan, let the chopped onion soften in the butter, place the floured veal shanks and let them color over high heat, salt and pepper. Pour the wine, let it evaporate, pour a little water, chopped celery and carrot, cook for half an hour. Add the tomato dissolved in a little water, stir and cook for another half hour.

Prepare the "gremolata": chop the peel of the lemon and a sprig of parsley, put the mixture on the veal shanks, warm up five minutes.

In a saucepan, heat 50 g of butter with the marrow, add the chopped onion and let it become transparent. Add the rice, mix it, wet it with a ladle of boiling broth and continue as for a normal risotto. Add salt. When the rice is al dente add the saffron dissolved in a little warm broth. Mix the risotto with the advanced butter and the grated cheese.

Place the shanks in the center of the plate and the risotto around. Bring to the table and serve immediately.

Enjoy your meal!

ORIENTAL GINGER MARINADE

Ingredients

5 cm of fresh ginger

Garlic cloves

2 lemons

1 bunch of coriander

1 teaspoon of garam masala

1 teaspoon of semi picante paprika

Preparation

Peel the ginger root and grate it (or mash it in a small garlic press). Put into a bowl, add the coriander leaves, the peeled and crushed garlic cloves, the paprika, the strained juice of the lemons and the garam masala (it is a mixture of powdered spices like cardamom, cinnamon, cloves, coriander, cumin). Stew for an hour.

Enjoy your meal!

AÏOLI SAUCE

Ingredients
3 cloves of garlic
1 yolk
1 lemon
1/2 glass of oil
Salt

Preparation
Peel the cloves of the garlic, place them in a bowl and mash them with a ladle. When they are reduced to a cream, add the yolk and, stirring, begin to slowly pour the oil like making mayonnaise. Complete with salt and lemon drops.
Enjoy your meal!

CLASSIC CITRONETTE

Ingredients for 4 people

4-5 tablespoons of oil
2 tablespoons of lemon juice
Salt

Preparation

Put the strained lemon juice and a pinch of salt in a bowl, stir for a few seconds with a small whisk or fork. Put the oil and continue to stir until you have a slightly opaque citronette.

Enjoy your meal!

MAYONNAISE

Ingredients for 4 people
2 egg yolks
About 2 dl of oil
1/2 lemon or 2 tablespoons of white vinegar
Salt and pepper

Preparation
Nowadays, mayonnaise is always sold and the market offers products on which you can rest assured. However, it is always useful to know how to do it by hand or with the blender, always use oil and eggs at the same room temperature (if too cold, mayonnaise may not "bind"); pour the oil in drops and the lemon or vinegar; if the mayonnaise "goes crazy" start all over again by mixing a new yolk with the crazy mixture poured drop by drop. By hand: put the egg yolks in a bowl, season with a pinch of salt and one of pepper. Then start pouring the oil drop by drop by mixing the ingredients with a small whisk. As soon as the mixture thickens, dilute it with a spray of lemon (or vinegar) and continue alternating oil and lemon until the mayonnaise is ready. With the blender: pour an egg yolk and a whole egg, salt, pepper, two tablespoons of oil and a little lemon juice into the glass. Blend for a few seconds at maximum speed. When the ingredients are mixed, add the remaining oil and lemon, blend for a minute. Adjust the salt. Pour into a sauce boat and keep in the fridge.
Enjoy your meal!

CUMBERLAND SAUCE

Ingredients for 4 people

2 oranges
2 lemons
2 tablespoons of mustard powder
2 tablespoons of currant jelly
2 tablespoons of red wine
2 tablespoons of vinegar
Salt
Pepper

Preparation

Cut the orange and the lemon peel into thin strips. If you use a normal knife avoid cutting the white skin underneath because it would make the sauce bitter. Blanch the fillets for 5 minutes, drain them. Squeeze the citrus fruits, collect the strained juice in a small saucepan, add the currant jelly, vinegar, wine, mustard, salt and pepper, bring to the boiling point. Then take it away, let the sauce cool, add the citrus fillets, mix well, serve in a sauce boat.
Enjoy your meal!

SALMORIGLIO SAUCE

Ingredients for 4 people
200 g of oil
2 lemons
Oregano
1 sprig of parsley
Salt
Pepper

Preparation
Put the oil into a bowl and beat it vigorously with the whisk. Add the strained lemon juice little by little, a tablespoon of hot water, the chopped parsley, a little oregano, salt and
pepper. This is a sauce that goes well with fish, especially with swordfish. If you want to use it for meat dishes you can replace the lemon with a little vinegar.
Enjoy your meal!

DESSERT

RICOTTA LEMON AND ALMOND DONUT

Ingredients for a donut mold with a diameter of 22 centimeters
3 whole eggs at room temperature
250 grams of cow's milk ricotta
150 grams of granulated sugar
1 packet of baking powder
The juice and peel of a grated lemon
50 grams of potato starch
100 grams of almonds or almond flour
200 grams of 00 flour
Flaked almonds for coverage

Preparation
Mix the ricotta with the sugar in a bowl.
When it is soft and creamy, add the eggs and continue stirring.
Add the peel and the juice of a lemon, the almond flour or chopped almonds and mix again.
Add the sifted potato starch and flour and finally the yeast sachet.
Pour the mixture into a donut-shaped mold, which is about 20/22 centimeters in diameter, sprinkle the surface of the cake with almond flakes and place it in a static oven, preheated to 180 ° for about 35 minutes. For the time and temperature, always adjust to your oven.
Enjoy your meal!

ANGELS' LEMON CAKE

Ingredients for a cake pan with a diameter of 22 centimeters
4 eggs at room temperature
150 grams of sugar
The juice and grated peel of a lemon
50 grams of chopped almonds
200 grams of 00 flour
150 grams of soft butter
1 package of baking powder
Icing sugar

Preparation
Melt the butter in a saucepan and let it cool.
Separate the yolks from the whites and whip them until they are stiff.
In a separate bowl whip the egg yolks with the granulated sugar, and when they are soft, add the butter and the chopped almonds.
Add the lemon juice and lemon peel and stir again.
Add the flour little by little (preferably sifted) and with the help of a spatula mix from the bottom upwards, add the yeast and stir again.
Finally, add the whipped egg whites to the mixture and pour everything into a buttered and floured cake pan.
Bake in a static oven, preheated to 180 ° for about 35-40 minutes, always adjust to your oven for the time and temperature. In any case, take the toothpick test.
Once cooked, let the cake cool well before removing it from the mold.
Sprinkle with plenty of icing sugar.
Enjoy your meal!

WATER DONUT WITH LEMON JUICE

Ingredients for a donut mold with a diameter of 22 centimeters
250 ml of warm water
150 ml of lemon juice
200 grams of sugar
350 grams of C0 flour
1 package of baking powder
100 ml of seed oil
Grated rind of a lemon
Icing sugar

Preparation
Put the water, lemon juice and the grated lemon peel in a bowl, add the sugar and stir until it is well dissolved.
Add the oil and stir again. Add the flour little by little, stirring constantly. Finally, add the yeast sachet as well.
Grease and flour the mold and pour the mixture.
Put the donut in a static oven, preheated to 180 ° for about 40 minutes. Always adjust to your own oven for the time and temperature. Do the toothpick test to see if the cake is cooked.
Let the cake cool. Before serving, sprinkle with plenty of icing sugar.
Enjoy your meal!

ALMOND AND LEMON DONUT

Ingredients for a 20 cm diameter mold
3 whole eggs at room temperature
200 grams of caster sugar (you can increase or decrease the amount as you like)
100 grams of peeled almonds
1 lemon
125 grams of plain yogurt
200 grams of flour
1 package of baking powder
Icing sugar

Preparation
First prepare the almond flour. Put the almonds and two tablespoons of sugar in the blender and blend. If you have a few pieces of almond left, leave them because you will use them for the dough.
Beat the eggs with the sugar. When the dough is soft and light, add the yogurt and stir. Then add the lemon juice and peel and the almond flour.
Add the flour and baking powder a little at a time.
Grease and flour the donut mold and pour the mixture.
Cook the cake in a static oven at 170 ° for about 30-35 minutes. Always adjust to your oven for the time and temperature.
Once cooked, let the donut cool before removing it from the mold.
Sprinkle the donut with icing sugar, and here it is in all its goodness, fragrant and light.
Enjoy your meal!

LEMON DONUT AND YOGURT

Ingredients

4 medium eggs at room temperature
150 grams of sugar
125 grams of plain yogurt or lemon
1 lemon
300 grams of 00 flour
1 package of baking powder
Icing sugar
Grains of sugar

Preparation

In a bowl mix the flour and the baking powder together and set aside. With an electric whisk or planetary mixer, whisk the eggs with sugar for at least 10 minutes. Add the yogurt a little at a time and stir gently with a spatula from the bottom upwards. Add the lemon juice and peel and stir.

Also sprinkle with flour and baking powder and mix by hand with the spatula from bottom to top.

Pour the mixture into a buttered and floured ring-shaped mold with a diameter of 24 centimeters. Sprinkle the surface with sugar granules and place the cake in a static oven at 170 ° for about 35-40 minutes. Always adjust to your oven for the time and temperature.

When the donut is puffed up and golden, place it on a plate and sprinkle with icing sugar.

Good, light, simple and fragrant, the lemon donut and yogurt is a dessert that everyone will like.

Enjoy your meal!

SOFT LEMON PLUMCAKE

Ingredients

3 medium eggs at room temperature
200 grams of granulated sugar
100 grams of potato starch
100 grams of 00 flour
250 grams of cow's milk ricotta
A package of baking powder
The juice and peel of a lemon
Grains of sugar to decorate

Preparation

With the planetary mixer or with the electric whisk, whisk the eggs with the sugar together at maximum speed. When the ricotta is puffed up and foamy, add the lemon juice and peel once the ricotta is well blended. Also add the starch, flour and finally the yeast sachet.

Grease and flour a plum cake mold and pour the mixture. Add the granulated sugar to the surface and place the cake in a static oven, preheated to 160 ° for about 35 minutes or until it is puffed up and golden. Remember to do the toothpick test if necessary: if it comes out clean it means it is cooked.

When the plumcake is cooked, leave it to cool before removing it from the mold.

The soft lemon plumcake is ready for your breakfasts or for welcoming a friend for tea time or a dessert for another time.

Enjoy your meal!

SHORTCRUST PASTRY

For the pastry

2 eggs

150 grams of sugar

150 grams of butter

400 grams of flour

For the custard

2 egg yolks

50 grams of flour or cornstarch

80 grams of sugar

200 ml of milk

Preparation

To prepare the pastry, place the flour on the pastry board. Add the egg yolks with the sugar and butter. Knead well until you have a soft and smooth dough. Let the pastry sit in the refrigerator until it is ready to be used.

Enjoy your meal!

LEMON CUSTARD

Ingredients for lemon cream
250 grams of water
150 grams of granulated sugar
50 grams of lemon juice
50 grams of butter
50 grams of potato starch
The grated rind of a lemon

Preparation
Put in a saucepan sugar, potato starch and lemon peel. Add the water and mix well. Put the mixture on the stove at a very low flame and stir constantly. After a few minutes the mixture will become gelatinous. At this point remove it from the heat and add the butter and lemon juice. Stir well until you have a smooth and velvet cream and let it cool. Make the cake.

Pour the lemon cream into the shortcrust and put the tart in the refrigerator for about 2 hours before serving. Decorate the lemon tart with meringues and lemon peel!

Enjoy your meal!

CHIFFON CAKE ROLLED WITH LEMON

Ingredients for chiffon cake
4 eggs at room temperature
150 grams of 00 flour
Half a bag of yeast
6 grams of tartar cream
The juice and grated peel of a lemon
100 grams of granulated sugar

For the cream
250 grams of ricotta
150 grams of mascarpone
50 grams of icing sugar
The juice and peel of half a lemon
Icing sugar for the cover

Preparation

Separate the yolks from the whites, beat the egg whites with half of the tartar cream and as soon as they begin to turn white add half of the sugar. Continue to stir them until they are well-blended. Separately, beat the egg yolks with the remaining sugar and when they are well mixed add the lemon juice and peel.

Gently add the egg yolks to the whites, stirring with a spatula from the bottom upwards.

Mix the yeast and the remaining tartar cream with the flour and add it little by little to the egg mixture. Pour the mixture on the baking tray covered with parchment paper cook it in a static oven, preheated to 150 ° for about 20-25 minutes. Always adjust to your oven for the times and temperature. Take it out when it's cooked. Put it on a damp cloth with all the parchment paper and roll it up while it is still warm, in this way it will take the form without breaking. In a bowl mix the ricotta, mascarpone, lemon and icing sugar. Take the roll, which now is completely cold, again and gently roll it out. Spread it with cream and roll it again leaving it wrapped in parchment paper. Refrigerate for at least two hours.

Enjoy your meal!

Tartar cream is a leavening agent, so it could be replaced with traditional baking powder, or with brewer's yeast. The tartar cream or fresh yeast is the same thing. In order to obtain the same leavening effect, it should be replaced with an ingredient that has a minimum acidity.

As natural acidifiers can be used: vinegar juice, lemon juice, sugar and egg whites.

When replacing the tartar cream you need to be very careful, because you will have to use the same amount of lemon, and for every millimeter of lemon or vinegar you'll have to add an egg white. To be able to replace it, and get the same effect, you have to whip the egg whites until stiff, this way it will give more softness to the cakes, or to sweet and savory dough.

If you are allergic or do not want to replace tartar cream with raising agents, you can choose to obtain the desired effect with a mixture of sparkling water and bicarbonate.

SOFT TART WITH WHITE CHOCOLATE AND LEMON CREAM

Ingredients for the pastry
300 grams of 00 flour
2 eggs
Half a bag of yeast
125 grams of granulated sugar
100 gram of butter
The peel of a grated lemon
100 grams of white chocolate
Icing sugar
Lemon peel

Preparation
Put the flour, eggs, butter, sugar, lemon zest and baking powder in a bowl. Mix everything well until you have a soft dough and let it rest in the fridge covered with a cloth.

Prepare the lemon cream and once it is ready, let it cool.

Take the soft pastry again and cover half of it with a hinged cake pan with a diameter of 20 centimeters. Also lift the edges well and pour the lemon cream.

In the remaining dough add the white chocolate in small pieces and put the mixture into the lemon cream until it is completely covered.

Put the cake in a static oven at 170 ° for about 45 minutes, always keeping in mind to adjust to your oven for the time and temperature.

When the tart is golden, remove it from the oven and let it cool well before removing it from the mold.

The soft tart with lemon cream and white chocolate is ready. Complete it with lemon peel and powdered sugar, it's a real treat!

Enjoy your meal!

SOFT LEMON CREAM CAKE

Ingredients for the cake

4 eggs at room temperature

200 grams of granulated sugar

125 grams of white yogurt and fruit yoghurt

The peel and the juice of a lemon

250 grams of 00 flour

1 package of baking powder

For the lemon cream

2 egg yolks

50 grams of corn flour or starch

The peel and the juice of a lemon

100 grams of granulated sugar

250 ml of milk

Preparation

First we must prepare the lemon cream: Put the milk in a saucepan to heat. In a bowl mix the egg yolks with the sugar and the flour, add the lemon juice and peel and stir. Pour the mixture in the hot milk and stir on a moderate heat until the cream becomes thick. Once the right consistency is reached, put the lemon cream to cool in a bowl.

Beat the eggs with the sugar at maximum speed. When they are puffed up and soft, add the lemon juice and peel. Add the flour and baking powder a little at a time.

Grease and flour a mold of 24 cm in diameter. First pour the mixture for the cake and then the cream by using a spoon. Put the cake in a static oven at 180 ° for about 40 minutes. Always adjust to your oven for the time and temperature.

When the cake is puffed up and golden, remove it from the oven and wait for it to cool well before removing it from the mold.

Serve the cake with lemon cream with plenty of icing sugar, a scent and a taste that will amaze you!

Enjoy your meal!

PUFF PASTRY SQUARES WITH LEMON CREAM

Ingredients

1 roll of puff pastry (preferably rectangular)
200 grams of custard
The juice and peel of a lemon
Icing sugar

Preparation

First prepare the custard and when it is ready add the lemon juice and peel. Stir and let it cool well. If you want to speed up the cooling process, place it into a bowl and put it in the fridge covered with cling film.

Take the puff pastry and spread it out on the work surface. Cut out squares of even numbers and pierce them with a fork. Put them on the baking paper in the baking tray of the oven and cook them at 170 ° in a static oven for about 10 minutes. Check them often because the puff pastry alone tends to darken quickly.

When the squares are golden brown, let them cool.

When the pastry squares have cooled, spread with cream to taste and overlap the other square of dough. Put them on a plate and sprinkle with plenty of icing sugar.

Serve the pastry squares with lemon cream for a snack, a delicious dessert, and also excellent as a dessert

if we have guests!

Enjoy your meal!

CUPCAKES WITH LEMON CREAM

Ingredients for 6 cupcakes
For the base
250 grams of biscuits (I used digestive, but normal biscuits are also good)
130 grams of melted butter
100 grams of lemon cream
50 grams of mascarpone or spreadable cheese

Preparation
For the base: Finely chop the biscuits, place them in a bowl and add the melted butter. Stir trying to get a compact dough.
Take some paper cups and in each one put a quantity of dough. With the back of a spoon or with your hand, mix the dough well in the baking cups, making them stick both on the bottom and on the walls of the baking cups. Once all the bases have been prepared, put them in the refrigerator for at least 30 minutes.
For the cream: Prepare the lemon cream, let it cool well and once cold, add the cream cheese you prefer. Stir with a spatula from the bottom upwards.
Take the bases of the cupcakes, gently remove them from the cups. Put them in a dish and in each one put a quantity of cream to taste and a slice of lemon. Put them back in the fridge until ready to serve.
Cakes with lemon cream are ready to be enjoyed!
Enjoy your meal!

CHEESECAKE ROLLS WITH LEMON CREAM

Ingredients for 4 rolls
2 slices of white bread without crust
200 grams of cream cheese
50 grams of granulated sugar
The juice and peel of half a lemon
1 egg
2 tablespoons of milk
Enough granulated sugar to cover
40 grams of butter

Preparation

Put the slices of bread on a cutting board and thin them lightly with a rolling pin. Cut them in half making 4 squares.
In a bowl mix the cream cheese with the sugar, the peel and the lemon juice.
Put a couple of tablespoons of cream on each slice of bread.
Roll the bread to obtain 4 rolls.
In a dish mix the egg with the milk and in another put the granulated sugar.
First, pass the rolls in the milk and egg mixture and then in the sugar.
Put them in a pan with the butter and let them brown for 5 minutes on each side on low heat.
They will be ready when they take on that golden color, we can serve them as soon as they are hot, but I recommend them lukewarm or even cold. The cheesecake rolls with lemon cream are a truly divine dessert!
Enjoy your meal!

LEMON AND MASCARPONE CREAM

Ingredients

3 lemons

3 egg yolks

120 grams of granulated sugar

30 grams of cornstarch or flour

30 grams of butter

100 ml of water

250 grams of mascarpone

50 grams of icing sugar

Preparation

Wash and dry the lemons. Grate the peel. Squeeze and put the juice and the grated peel in a saucepan, add the water and light the flame very low. While the juice warms, in a dish beat the egg yolks with the sugar and cornstarch or flour. Remove the liquid of water and lemon from the heat, add the butter, stir until completely dissolved and then pour in the egg mixture. Light the fire which will always be low and stir until completely thickened. Pour the lemon cream (which is already so good) in a bowl and let it cool well. Put the mascarpone in a bowl with the icing sugar and mix it until it is becomes soft. Pour the lemon cream into the mascarpone and mix everything well.

Put the cream in the fridge for a couple of hours.

Enjoy your meal!

CREAMY LEMON CAKE

Ingredients

4 Eggs (at room temperature)
100 g Fecola Di Patate (or corn starch)
100 g of 00 flour
3 Lemons (both the juice and the peel)
250 g Ricotta Vaccina
80 g Butter (melted)
20 g Coconut Flour
Baked Powder Yeast (1 sachet)
150 g Sugar

Preparation

First you need to prepare the lemon juice. Scrub the peel first, taking care not to add the white part of the lemon, also squeeze the juice of all the lemons and set aside. Sift all the powders together; then flour, starch and yeast and keep these aside in a bowl. In a bowl and with the help of a whisk, make the ricotta creamy together with the sugar, add the eggs, one at a time, when the previous egg is well mixed together with the next one. Add the melted butter (not boiling) and the lemon juice and peel.

Also add the powders (flour, yeast and starch) and coconut flour. Mix with a spatula and pour the mixture into a buttered and floured cake pan with a diameter of 24 centimeters. Cook the cake in a static oven at 170 ° for about 35 minutes. Always adjust to your oven for the time and temperature. Once the cake is golden and has made a crust, take it out of the oven and let it cool.

Enjoy your meal!

LEMON PIE

Ingredients for lemon cream

250 grams of water
150 grams of granulated sugar
50 grams of lemon juice
50 grams of butter
50 grams of potato starch
The grated rind of a lemon
To decorate: meringues, lemon peel

Preparation
For the base

First prepare the pastry, wrap it in plastic wrap and let it rest for about half an hour. When it has rested, roll out the pastry and spread it in a mold for pies with a diameter of 20 centimeters. Cover the pastry base with a sheet of parchment paper and dried beans and cook in a static oven at 180 ° for about 25 minutes. When cooked, place it gently on a plate to cool.

For the lemon cream

Put in a saucepan sugar, potato starch and lemon peel. Add the water and mix well. Put the mixture on the gas at a very low flame and stir constantly. After a few minutes the mixture will become gelatinous, at this point remove it from the heat and add the butter and lemon juice. Stir well until you have a smooth and velvet cream and let it cool. Make the cake.

Pour the lemon cream into the shortcrust base and put the tart in the refrigerator for about 2 hours before serving. Decorate the lemon tart with meringues and lemon peel!

Enjoy your meal!

LEMON BISCUITS WITHOUT BUTTER

Ingredients
3 egg yolks
250 grams of flour
120 grams of sugar
The peel of half a lemon
50 ml of peanut or sunflower oil
A pinch of salt
A pinch of yeast (just under half a teaspoon)
Lemon cream (see recipe in the book)

Preparation
First prepare the lemon cream and let it cool well.
For the lemon cream
Put in a saucepan sugar, potato starch and lemon peel. Add the water and mix well. Put the mixture on the gas at a very low flame and stir constantly. After a few minutes the mixture will become gelatinous, at this point remove it from the heat and add the butter and lemon juice. Stir well until you have a smooth and velvet cream and let it cool.
Knead on a pastry board or in a bowl, the flour with the eggs, the grated peel of half a lemon, the oil, the sugar, the salt and the yeast and form a soft dough.
Take a piece of pastry of about 25 grams each with your hands and form a dome and place them on a baking sheet lined with parchment paper well spaced from one another. With your finger, press lightly in the center of each cookie.
Put them in a static oven, preheated to 180 ° for about 20 minutes, for the time and temperature always adjust to your oven.
Once cooked, let them cool well.
Use your finger to press lightly on each cookie and fill with lemon cream.
Lemon biscuits without butter are ready to be enjoyed.
Enjoy your meal!

LEMON CHEESECAKE SQUARES IN PUFF PASTRY

Ingredients

1 pack of frozen puff pastry (inside you will find 2 rolls) or 2 rolls of a fresh one
500 grams of cream cheese
100 grams of ricotta
1 lemon both peel and juice
100 grams of icing sugar
Icing sugar for the cover
Melted butter
Caster sugar

Preparation

Mix the cream cheese and ricotta well in a bowl. Add the icing sugar, lemon juice and peel, and stir.

Unroll the puff pastry and cover a rectangular pan with a sheet of parchment paper. Cover it with the first roll, prick the base, pour the cream cheese and cover with the other roll of pastry trying to seal the edges well.

Brush the surface with melted butter and add a handful of granulated sugar. Cook the cake in a static oven at 170 ° for about 15 minutes and when it is golden brown remove it from the oven and let it cool in its mold at room temperature. Place it in the refrigerator for about 2 hours.

Cut the meal into squares and sprinkle with icing sugar.

They are delicate, very fresh and so fragrant!

Enjoy your meal!

LEMON AND WHITE CHOCOLATE CHEESECAKE WITHOUT COOKING

Ingredients
For the base
200 grams of biscuits (you can also use other biscuits)
150 grams of butter
For the cream
400 grams of mascarpone or philadelphia
350 grams of whipping cream
100 grams of icing sugar
10 grams of isinglass as an alternative to natural agar agar
100 grams of white chocolate
The juice and peel of a lemon

Preparation
Finely chop the biscuits and place them into a bowl. Add the melted butter and mix well. Cover a 22 cm diameter mold with parchment paper and pour the crumbled biscuits. Press them down with the back of a spoon and place the base in the refrigerator.

Whip the cream with the icing sugar and add the mascarpone cheese a little at a time. Soften the gelatin in cold water, squeeze it and melt it in a little hot milk. Add it to the cream, taking it through a sieve. Also add the lemon peel and juice to the cream and divide the mixture into two bowls. Melt the white chocolate and add it to one of the two bowls and mix well. Take the biscuit base and pour the white cream. Level and leave in the fridge for about 15-20 minutes. When it is thickened, pour the white chocolate cream and level again. Let the cake rest in the fridge for at least 3 hours.

Serve the lemon and white chocolate cheesecake with chocolate curls and lemon zest, which will melt in your mouth!

Enjoy your meal!

TART WITH RICOTTA AND LEMON CREAM

Ingredients

For the base

300 grams of pastry, my recipe HERE

For the stuffing

300 grams of cow ricotta

50 grams of icing sugar

200 grams of lemon cream for the recipe click HERE

For coverage

Icing sugar

Preparation

Prepare the pastry and let it rest in the refrigerator.

Also prepare the lemon cream and let it cool very well. In a bowl mix the cow ricotta with the icing sugar making it creamy (I always choose cow ricotta for my desserts because I don't like that of sheep, because it is too strong, but if you like it you can use it easily).

Take the pastry again and spread out a circle about half a centimeter on the pastry board with the help of a rolling pin. Grease and flour a tart mold with a diameter of 20 cm and line it with the pastry. Prick the base and pour the ricotta. Level well and pour the lemon cream on the ricotta. Finish the tart with the classic strips and bake it in a static oven, preheated to 180° for about 35 minutes. When it is golden, let it cool very well before removing it from the mold. Serve the tart with ricotta and lemon cream with a sprinkling of icing sugar.

Enjoy your meal!

GIRELLE WITH LEMON CREAM AND WHITE CHOCOLATE

Ingredients

2 slices of soft bread without crust
120 grams of lemon cream my recipe HERE
100 grams of white chocolate

Preparation

Take the slices of bread and place them on top of each other. Thin them slightly with a rolling pin. Spread the lemon cream evenly and roll the bread, wrap it in a sheet of parchment paper and leave it in the fridge for about 1 hour so that the circles are easier to cut. Melt the white chocolate in a bain-marie or in the microwave.

Take the roll from the refrigerator and cut about 4 cm circls. Dip half of them in the melted chocolate and place them on a sheet of parchment paper with the part covered in chocolate facing upwards. Leave them in the fridge just long enough to solidify the white chocolate. Serve the Girelle with lemon cream and white chocolate for a snack, but they are also suitable for parties and buffets.

Enjoy your meal!

LEMON CHEESECAKE BROWNIES SWEET RECIPE

Ingredients

For the base of the lemon brownies

2 eggs at room temperature

60 grams of melted butter

200 grams of 00 flour

Half a teaspoon of yeast

100 grams of granulated sugar

The juice and peel of half a lemon

For the cream

120 grams of cow's milk ricotta

250 grams of philadelphia (or spreadable cheese)

120 grams of sugar

The juice and peel of half a lemon

5 grams of isinglass or agar agar which is a natural thickener and is found in all supermarkets

3 tablespoons of warm milk

Preparation

Beat the eggs with the sugar. Add the lemon juice and peel, flour, baking powder and melted butter, mix well and pour the mixture into a 20 x 20 square baking sheet covered with parchment paper. Cook the base in a static oven, preheated to 170 ° for about 20 minutes, in the meantime prepare the cream. Put the ricotta in a bowl with the philadelphia (or spreadable cheese) and the sugar. Add the lemon juice and peel and mix well.

Put the isinglass in cold water and when it is soft squeeze it. Melt it in hot milk and add it to the cream, filtering it through a sieve. When the base is cooked, let it cool. Pour the cream on the cold base and level. Refrigerate at least 2 hours before serving. Serve the lemon cheesecake brownies cut into squares, fresh and delicious.

Enjoy your meal!

LEMON RICE DONUT (LIGHT DESSERT RECIPE)

Ingredients

4 eggs

150 grams of granulated sugar

200 grams of rice flour

1 lemon

100 ml of milk

Yeast sachet

50 ml of seed oil

Icing sugar

Preparation

Whisk the eggs with the sugar for 10 minutes. When they are soft and fluffy, add the oil and milk and mix again. Add the lemon juice and grated peel.

Add the rice flour a little at a time and gently mix the mixture with a spatula, then add the yeast. Pour the mixture into a donut-shaped mold with a diameter of 26 cm. Cook the cake in a static oven, preheated to 180 ° for about 30 minutes, always adjusting to your oven. The Rice Donut will be ready when you see it golden and swollen, at this point remove it from the oven and let it cool well before removing it from the mold.

Serve the Lemon Rice Donut with plenty of icing sugar.

Enjoy your meal!

MASCARPONE WITH LEMON AND WHITE CHOCOLATE

Ingredients
100 grams of granulated sugar (you can increase or decrease depending on the taste)
Icing sugar to decorate

Preparation

Mix the flour with the egg, the baking powder, the sugar and the butter in a bowl. Knead vigorously with your hand but not too much, the desired effect is for it to be crumbled. In a separate bowl mix the ricotta with the sugar and the lemon juice. Add the grated lemon peel and stir again. Take a 22 cm diameter cake pan and cover it with a sheet of parchment paper. Put half the dough on the base and press down well. Add the ricotta and lemon cream and complete the cake with the other dough, crumble over the cream with your hands. Cook in a preheated static oven at 170 ° for about 25 minutes. Always adjust to your oven.

Serve the mascarpone with ricotta cream and lemon with a sprinkling of icing sugar. Keep the cake in the fridge for up to 3 days.

Enjoy your meal!

NEW YORK LEMON CHEESECAKE

Ingredients

For the base

250 grams of digestive biscuits

120 grams of butter

For the cream

500 grams of philadelphia

2 egg yolks + 1 whole egg

200 grams of sugar

The grated rind of 2 lemons

The juice of 1 lemon

2 teaspoons of cornstarch

For the icing

70 grams of icing sugar

The juice of 1 lemon

1 teaspoon of honey

Preparation

First, cover a 22 cm diameter hinge mold with parchment paper. Finely chop the biscuits and add the melted butter. Mix well and pour everything into the mold. Press the base well and try to make a border with the biscuits. Let it rest in the refrigerator and in the meantime prepare the cream. Put the philadelphia (or spreadable cheese) and the sugar in the planetary mixer and whisk until becomes creamy. Add the egg yolks one at a time, and the whole egg too. Add the peel of the lemons and also the juice.

Take the base out of the fridge and pour the cream over the biscuits. Level well and place the cake in a preheated static oven at 170 ° for about 50 minutes, the time and temperature depends on your oven. Check the cheesecake often and when it has a golden crust it means that it is ready. Remove it from the oven and let it cool at room temperature in its mold for at least 2 hours. Then put the mold in the fridge for another 2-3 hours. Prepare a glaze by putting lemon juice with honey and icing sugar in a saucepan. Stir but don't boil. Take out the New York lemon cheesecake from the fridge. Put it on a plate, pour the lemon icing over the cake and serve it while it's cold.

Enjoy your meal!

COLD CAKE WITH LEMON AND RICOTTA (RECIPE WITHOUT COOKING)

Ingredients
For the base
250 grams of frollini biscuits
120 grams of butter
For the cream
600 grams of cow's milk ricotta
150 grams of sugar
8 grams of isinglass
The juice and peel of 1 lemon
For coverage
4 grams of isinglass
The juice of half a lemon
100 ml of water
3 tablespoons of sugar
A few drops of yellow food coloring

Preparation
Crumble the biscuits and add the melted butter. Mix well until the two ingredients are mixed together. Cover a 22 cm diameter hinge mold with parchment paper and cover the bottom with the biscuits. Press the biscuits to make them stick together and press them down well at the bottom of the mold. Put them in the refrigerator for about 30 minutes.

Sift the ricotta, add the sugar and the lemon juice and peel and work with the electric whisk until it is creamy. Put the gelatine sheets in cold water, squeeze and melt it in a little hot liquid, it's good to have a little milk or water. Add it to the ricotta through a sieve, stir and pour everything on the biscuit base.

Put the cake in the refrigerator and in the meantime prepare the cover. Put the isinglass in cold water. Put the 100 ml of water, the lemon juice and the sugar in a saucepan and let it heat on a low heat. Remove the water from the heat and add the isinglass. Mix it very well until it is well dissolved and also add a few drops of yellow dye to give it the cheerful and lively color of the lemon. Pour the gelatine on the cake and let it rest in the refrigerator for at least 3 hours. The cold cake with lemon and ricotta is ready to be enjoyed. Enjoy your meal!

QUICK DONUTS WITH RICOTTA AND LEMON

Ingredients

300 g flour

125 g Ricotta Vaccina

1 Eggs

100 g Sugar (you can increase to 150 if you want a sweeter result)

1 Lemon (both the juice and the grated peel)

8 g Yeast Powder For Sweets

Q.s. Peanut Oil

Q.s. Sugar (for coverage)

Preparation

In a large bowl pour the flour (preferably sifted first) in the center and add: the egg, the ricotta, the juice and the peel of the lemon, the sugar, and the yeast. Mix all the ingredients with a spoon to mix them together and then with your hand to form a soft dough.

Put the dough on a lightly floured pastry board and spread a circle about half a centimeter thick. With a pasta bowl (I used one of 5 cm) make circles and in each circle make a hole in the center. Heat plenty of oil in a fry and dip the donuts maximum 3/4 at a time, otherwise you risk lowering the oil temperature. Cook and brown them on both sides turning them often.

When the donuts with ricotta and lemon are puffed up and golden, drain them on kitchen paper to absorb the excess oil and pass them in the granulated sugar while they are still warm. Serve it during breakfast!

Enjoy your meal!

COLD LEMON AND WHITE CHOCOLATE CAKE WITH DOUBLE BISCUIT

Ingredients
For biscuit bases
300 grams of crumbly biscuits
120 grams of melted butter
For the white cream
120 grams of icing sugar
250 grams of cream
250 grams of mascarpone or philadephia
50 grams of white chocolate
8 grams of isinglass (as a replacement you can use agar agar which is found in organic stores)
2 tablespoons of warm milk
For the lemon yellow cream
2 lemons
2 egg yolks
50 grams of butter
1 tablespoon of cornstarch
70 grams of sugar
To decorate: slices of lemon, white chocolate

Preparation
For the base: with the help of a food procesor, crush the biscuits into fine crumbs, add the melted butter to the biscuits and mix very well. Cover a cake pan with a diameter of 24 cm that can with parchment paper. Pour half of the biscuits (the other half will serve later) and press well with a spoon to make them stick to the bottom. Put the base in the refrigerator.
For the lemon cream: squeeze two lemons and collect the juice in a saucepan. Also add 3 tablespoons of water, the butter and put on the gas at a very low flame. In a dish, mix the egg yolks with the sugar and cornstarch, remove the pan from the heat and pour the egg yolks, stirring constantly. Put on low heat and turn with a wooden spoon until it thickens. Cool the lemon cream well.

For the white cream: whip the cream with the sugar and add the mascarpone or philadelphia, depending on your choice. Mix very well from the bottom upwards and also add the white chocolate crushed into small pieces. Soak the isinglass, squeeze it and let it dissolve in two tablespoons of warm milk and add it to the cream. Return the biscuit base to the refrigerator. Pour all the white cream, leveling well. Pour the other half of the biscuits we kept aside and spread them with a wet spatula on the white cream. Also pour the lemon custard on the biscuits and level well. Put the cake in the refrigerator at least 3-4 hours.

Enjoy your meal!

LEMON AND WHITE CHOCOLATE PARFAIT

Ingredients

250 ml of fresh cream

125 grams of icing sugar

2 egg yolks

2 lemons

200 ml of milk

70 grams of sugar

30 grams of flour

100 grams of white chocolate

Preparation

To prepare the lemon cream, heat the milk on a low flame. Place the egg yolks, the juice and the rind of 1 lemon, the flour and the sugar in a dish. Mix everything and pour into the hot milk. Mix the cream with a wooden spoon until it thickens. Turn off the heat and let it cool very well.

Whip the cream with the icing sugar and the grated rind of the other lemon. Take a plumcake mold, cover it with plastic wrap and pour half of the whipped cream on the bottom. Level and add a layer of lemon cream, cover the lemon cream with another layer of cream and put everything in the freezer for about 2 hours.

After 2 hours, melt the white chocolate, remove the semifreddo from the mold, place it on a plate and pour over the white chocolate trying to cover it all. Let the chocolate firm up for a few minutes and serve

Enjoy your meal!

LEMON MERINGUE

Ingredients
For the pastry
2 eggs
150 grams of sugar
150 grams of butter
400 grams of flour
For the custard
2 egg yolks
50 grams of flour or cornstarch
80 grams of sugar
200 ml of milk
For the lemon cream
2 egg yolks
Juice and peel of 2 lemons
1 tablespoon of cornstarch
100 grams of sugar
70 grams of butter
For the meringue
3 egg whites
120 grams of sugar
A few drops of lemon

Preparation

To prepare the pastry: place the flour on the pastry board, add the egg yolks with the sugar and the butter and knead well until you have a soft and smooth dough. Let the pastry stand in the refrigerator until it is ready to be used.

For the custard: heat the milk in a saucepan. In a dish, beat the egg yolks with the sugar and cornstarch. Add the hot milk a little at a time and transfer everything to the pan. Mix well until it thickens. When it has reached the right consistency put it into a bowl and let it cool.

For the lemon cream: in a saucepan put the lemon juice with the grated peel, the butter and let it melt. Beat the eggs with the sugar and add them with lemon and butter. Stir on low heat until it thickens.

When both creams are cold, blend them together, mixing well.

Put in a kneader (the kneader would be the best choice but you can also do it with a blender) the egg whites with sugar and a few drops of lemon and mix at maximum speed. At this point we can assemble the dessert. Take a tart mold of 26 cm in diameter and make a pastry. Put it in the pan and pierce the base with a fork. Add the cream and finally the meringue.

For the meringue: cook the lemon meringue pie in a preheated oven at 170 degrees for about 25 minutes. When it is almost cooked, turn on the grill for about 5 minutes. When it is cooked, let it cool and keep in the fridge for at least a few hours before eating it.

Enjoy your meal!

LEMON DONUT WITH RICOTTA (RECIPE WITHOUT BUTTER)

Ingredients

4 eggs
100 grams of granulated sugar
4 tablespoons of wildflower honey
250 grams of 00 flour
40 ml of milk
1 packet of yeast
250 grams of cow's milk ricotta

For the lemon icing

1 egg white
125 grams of icing sugar
The juice of 1 lemon

Preparation

In a kneader basket (or blender if you do not have the kneader) put the eggs with the sugar and honey and whisk at maximum speed for about 10 minutes. Add the ricotta and milk, lowering the speed. Add the flour a little at a time and gently mix it with a spatula from the bottom upwards. Add the yeast and pour it into a donut mold with a diameter of 26 cm. Cook the cake in a static oven at 160 ° for about 35-40 minutes, doing the toothpick test because every oven has its own power. When it is cooked, take the donut out of the oven and let it cool well.

For the icing: in a bowl, mix the egg white with the lemon juice and the icing sugar and pour everything into a saucepan. Let it heat on a low flame stirring constantly and when it becomes white, remove it from the heat. Pour the icing on the donut. Let it set a little before serving. If you want, you can decorate the lemon donut with lemon zest.

Enjoy your meal!

LEMON CAKE WITH RICOTTA AND PINE NUTS

Ingredients

4 eggs
The juice and peel of 2 lemons
125 g of cow's milk ricotta
20 g of pine nuts
150 grams of granulated sugar
300 gr of 00 flour
1 packet of yeast
Icing sugar for cover.

Preparation

In the planetary mixer put the eggs with the sugar and whip them until they are soft. Add the ricotta, reducing the speed, the juice, the lemon rind and the flour a little at a time. Grease and flour a mold with a diameter of 24 cm and pour the mixture, leveling well. Sprinkle the surface of the cake with pine nuts and a icing sugar. Put it in the oven at 180 ° for about 25-30 minutes. Serve the lemon cake with ricotta and pine nuts when it is very cold and for a sweet tooth may be accompanied by a custard.
Enjoy your meal!

LEMON CAKE WITH PHILADELPHIA CREAM

Ingredients
For the cake
4 eggs
350 g of 00 flour
200 grams of sugar
50 ml of sunflower oil
1 package of yeast
For the cream
1 egg + 1 yolk
120 grams of sugar
150 ml of milk
3 tablespoons of cornstarch
3 tablespoons of philadelphia or spreadable cheese
The juice and peel of 1 lemon
Icing sugar q.b.

Preparation

Whisk the eggs with the sugar for at least 10 minutes. Add the oil and gradually add the flour and finally the yeast sachet. Pour everything into a cake pan with a diameter of 24 cm and cook the cake in a preheated oven at 180 ° for about 35 minutes. When it is cooked, let it cool well. While the base is cooling down, start preparing the cream. Put the egg, the yolk and the sugar in a bowl and mix well with a whisk. Add the lemon juice, the cornstarch and the previously heated milk. Put everything in a saucepan and thicken the cream on low heat, stirring constantly. When the cream has reached the right consistency put it into a bowl and let it cool. When it is cold, add the philadelphia or other spreadable cheese. Mix well. Take the base and cut it in half. Spread with cream and cover with the other disk. Sprinkle the cake with lemon and philadelphia cream with plenty of icing sugar and store it in the refrigerator before serving.
Enjoy your meal!

HOMEMADE LIMONCELLO

Ingredients
700 ml of water
500 ml of 95 ° alcohol
500 g (about 6) of untreated lemon
600 g of sugar

Preparation
Carefully wash the organic lemons and dry them with a cloth. Peel the lemons with a vegetable peeler, taking care not to remove the white part because it is bitter. Cut the rind into small pieces, preferably using a ceramic knife.

Pour the pure alcohol in an airtight container along with the lemon zest reduced to small pieces. Leave the lemon peel in the container for 3 weeks, taking care to turn the container often to facilitate the extraction of the active ingredients.

After 3 weeks, proceed with the preparation of the syrup. Bring the water to the boiling point and melt the sugar. Let it cool completely. Add the cooled syrup to the alcohol and lemon peel. Leave to macerate for another 7 days. Filter the liqueur from the lemon peel (which in the meantime will have yielded most of the active ingredients), bottled and served iced. The limoncello can be kept in the freezer: the alcohol and sugar contained inside prevent it from freezing.

Considering that the active ingredients contained in the lemon are photosensitive and thermolabile (sensitive to light and heat) it is recommended to wrap the glass container with aluminum foil, or to prefer a dark glass container. For the same reason, it is advisable to store alcohol with lemon peel in a cool environment, away from heat sources.

Enjoy your meal!

LEMON SORBET WITHOUT ICE CREAM MAKER

Ingredients for 6 people

500 ml of water

200 grams of sugar

180 ml of lemon juice

The rind of half a lemon

Preparation

Clean the lemons in the inner part without damaging the outer skin: they will serve as cups to contain the sorbet.

Melt the sugar and water in a saucepan on a very low heat until it forms a syrup. Remove from the heat and let it cool.

Add the lemon juice and the grated rind. Put it in the ice containers and leave it in the freezer for 12 hours.

Put the cubes in the blender or food processor and operate at maximum speed until a thick cream is obtained.

Pour the sorbet into the emptied lemons. Do the same procedure to prepare sorbet with other types of fruit.

Enjoy your meal!

LEMON MOUSSE

Ingredients

Lemon juice 60 ml
Gelatin in sheets 10 g
Fresh liquid cream 400 ml
Sugar 250 g
Egg whites (about 4 medium eggs) 150 g

Preparation

Put a thick bottomed pot on fire. Pour the lemon juice, 150 grams of sugar and melt on low heat until the sugar has completely melted; the syrup should not exceed 121 ° C, you can measure with a kitchen thermometer.

When it reaches the temperature of 116 ° C, start beating the egg whites with the mixer or planetary at medium speed. The mixture should turn white after which add the remaining sugar. When the syrup reaches 121 ° and at the same time the egg whites are well whipped, pour it on the egg whites, continuing to beat them at medium speed; let the whips go until the mixture is completely cold. Once ready, you will get an Italian meringue that will have a white and frothy consistency. Once the meringue is ready put it aside and in the meantime soak the gelatin in sheets into a bowl with cold water for at least 10 minutes.

Heat 50 ml of cream in a saucepan and when it is hot add the squeezed gelatine sheets. Mix with a whisk to completely melt the gelatine. Then turn off the heat and let it cool. Separately, whip the remaining cream.

Then add the cream in which you have dissolved the isinglass to the meringue, by now cold and gently mix everything. Let it rest in the refrigerator for 2 hours.

After two hours, remove the lemon mousse from the fridge and pour it into a sac-à-poche. Fill the cups to the brim. Serve the mousse with almond biscuits!

Enjoy your meal!

LEMON GRANITA WITHOUT ICE CREAM MAKER

Ingredients
Lemon juice 500 ml
Water 500 ml
Sugar 250 g

Preparation
To prepare the lemon granita without ice cream maker, pour the water into a saucepan, bring it to the boiling point and add the sugar. When the sugar has completely melted and the liquid has become transparent, turn off the heat and whisk the mixture. At this point, put the lemon granita in the freezer inside a plastic (metal) covered container. After half an hour, take the mixture out of the freezer and stir it vigorously to break the ice crystals that have formed. Repeat the same operation every half an hour (or every quarter of an hour if you see that the mixture tends to compact faster) for another two or three times, until you get the lemon granita without ice cream maker of the desired consistency.
Enjoy your meal!

Thanks again for choosing this book, make sure to leave a short review on Amazon if you enjoy it. I'd really love to hear your thoughts!

If you don't like the book, send me an email to deltonevo@gmail.com with your suggestions to improve it!

Conclusion

In conclusion, lemon does lead to weight loss, but along with healthy eating and exercising. It is known that the difficulty of losing weight lies in a slow digestive system. If you are going to drink water with lemon for weight loss, you will need to drink 8-10 200 ml glasses a day and once you lose weight continue drinking. You will need to eat at least five servings of fruit and vegetables, five or six small meals every day and eliminate the foods that cotain sugar. You will have to eat the right fats. Unsaturated fats actually help lose weight because they delay the entry of carbohydrates into the bloodstream. You will also have to consume omega and omega 6 which can be found in: nuts, seeds and fish oil. You will have to consume many whole and fresh foods such as whole wheat pasta, whole grains, vegetables, fruit, fresh soups, smoothies, salad with every meal. You will need to limit all alcohol-based drinks. Allow yourself only half a glass of wine a day and limit your consumption of coffee and tea. You will need to avoid carbonated drinks and sugary fruit juices. When you eat fruit, you should also eat a handful of nuts or seeds to help slow the impact of natural sugars on the body. Avoid artificial sweeteners and saturated fats.

Another important thing for a healthy digestive system and weight loss is to eat slowly. Nowadays, because of our frenetic society, we tend to eat so fast that we do not taste what we eat. Take the time to chew properly, because the chewing process serves more than one purpose. It relaxes the lower stomach muscles and sends nerve impulses to activate the digestive process. If you do not take the time to chew your food thoroughly, the nutrients are not digested.

Portion control is another key factor for losing weight. Eat moderate portions and if you think you want more wait 20 minutes. This gives the brain time to get in touch with the stomach to see if you are really still hungry or not.

If you drink water with lemon to lose weight and follow the other guidelines of the lemon juice diet you do not have to worry about counting calories. Recommended foods can be eaten at will (but remember to wait 20 minutes to make sure you if are really hungry). Drink water and lemon in at least one meal a day. Also, exercise 30 minutes a day at least five days in a week and you will see how you lose weight.

A good option to obtain even better results is to consume lemon with green tea. By adding the precious citrus fruit to green tea, you will be confident enough to be able to stimulate weight loss discreetly and consciously. It is known that green tea with lemon represents a winning element in any path of weight loss and it seems that taking at least 4 glasses of green tea a day can double the effectiveness of any weight loss procedure. In short, a real sensational mix to ensure all the typical benefits of this drink.

As obvious, in conclusion of this brief study, our suggestion is of course not to overdo the intake of water and lemon, since even in this case the excess could harm. Before embarking on any weight loss program and modifying your diet, talk about it with your doctor, who will certainly be able to explain to you what to do to achieve the goals you have set without necessarily having to go to unbalance your eating habits. Do-it-yourself can be a good temptation but it is often better to let it go.